IMPROVING CONCENTRATION

Evaluating and improving concentration and performance

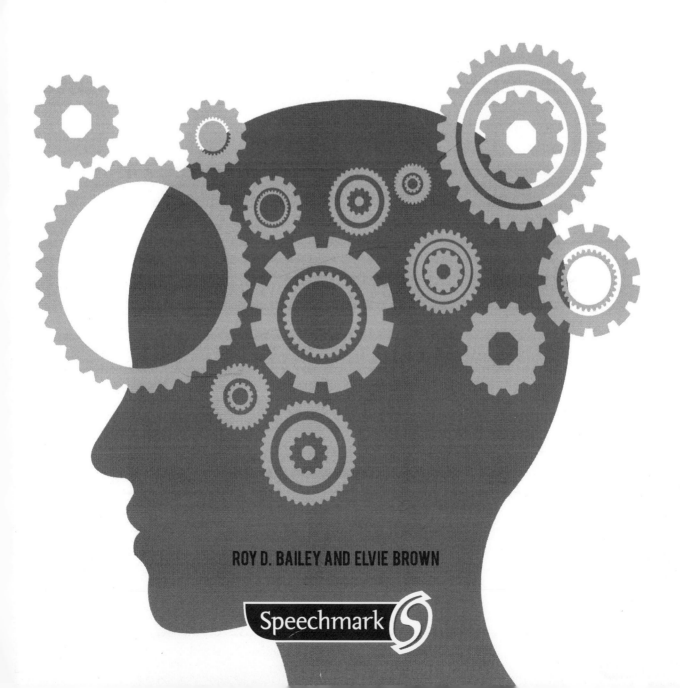

ROY D. BAILEY AND ELVIE BROWN

Speechmark

First published in 2015 by
Speechmark Publishing Ltd,
St Mark's House, Shepherdess Walk, London N1 7BQ, United Kingdom
www.speechmark.net

002-5787 Printed in the United Kingdom by CMP (uk) Ltd

Design and artwork by Moo Creative (Luton)

British Library Cataloguing in Publication Data
A catalogue record for this book is available from the British Library

ISBN: 978 0 86388 910 3

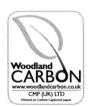

CONTENTS

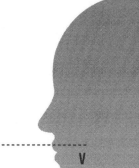

We learn many things in our formal education and lifetime. Unfortunately, learning how to concentrate is not one of them.

(Bailey, 2012)

PREFACE

The motivation to produce this resource arose from an increasing number of referrals for psychological assessment and calls for assistance where the main cause for concern was an individual's concentration difficulties. It soon emerged that some of these people were aware that impaired concentration was an issue for them. Others simply believed, or were told, they 'could not concentrate'. Beyond this, they had little or no insight into the nature of their difficulties or how to bring about any desirable change. The general assumption held by many was that, although concentration issues were the cause of many of their performance difficulties, they could not be understood or changed.

In this resource, we show you why we do not accept this position. Recent developments in neuroscience suggest that the brain can be altered by reprogramming areas of it to perform better and so aid concentration. More recently, mindfulness training techniques have also been shown to produce fundamental changes in neurological processes. These are exciting developments because they suggest that, wherever there is a connection between brain function and performance, we may find ways of influencing neurological processes to the advantage of the individual (Brown & Bailey, 2012; Fehemi & Robbins, 2007).

The message is clear. We can help people to better understand their concentration difficulties, learn concentration skills and improve their ability to concentrate.

INTRODUCTION

Who is this resource for?

Improving Concentration has been designed to help individuals improve their concentration skills. It is aimed primarily at the people with a training role in relation to the individual concerned. However, the individuals themselves can also use it as a self-help resource.

This resource will help trainers to convey to their students:

1 an understanding of concentration
2 how concentration works for them
3 how the student can improve their concentration skills
4 how the student can manage concentration in relation to their performance.

How to use *Improving Concentration*

This psychological skills training resource is arranged to be both easy to use and clear to follow. The activities can be used with both individual students and groups. There are three parts as follows.

Part 1 'Understanding concentration' outlines the theoretical perspectives on concentration and describes the Bailey and Brown model of concentration. Trainers can use Part 1 to increase their own conceptual understanding of the topic. This knowledge base can then be conveyed to their students when it is appropriate.

Part 2 'Pathways to improving concentration' explains and describes how the Bailey and Brown model of concentration can be used as a guide to raising awareness, understanding, monitoring and evaluating interventions aimed at improving concentration in people. Part 2 also outlines a mindful approach to coaching. We suggest how mindful coaching can be used with people to facilitate their awareness, attention, openness, curiosity, patience and thinking, to create new choices and behaviours that can improve their concentration.

Part 3 'Concentration skills training' contains a range of activities. This part of the resource can be used either alone or as part of a structured intervention to improve an individual's concentration skills. The purpose of each activity is outlined, and the specific additional resources needed are listed. Each activity is related to the model of concentration and the trainer can choose activities according to the student's specific areas of difficulty.

A Concentration Activities Guide (CAG) is included to assist you in selecting and designing training interventions. Each improving concentration activity gives you an explanation of how to proceed and how to review performance.

Materials

Marker pens and pencils

Keep plenty of pens and pencils available. They are useful for emphasising key points and may be needed at any point during an activity.

Computer technology

Where possible, computer aids can help with recording and providing further information to the student. Notepads or laptops can be used either to enhance learning or as a recording device.

Flipcharts

A flipchart can still be a useful teaching aid for the trainer. It can be used interactively with students or it can provide a flexible way of enhancing topic information.

Notebooks or personal journals

It is important to have a form of recording information from a training session. Some of the activities include space for making notes. In any event, a system of retaining the activities for each student will be necessary, for example in a personal folder.

Some students may prefer to make computer-based notes for themselves. They will still need a folder in which to keep their own specific record of the activities they have done. The trainer will also need to keep their own record of the activities completed with the student and notes about the student's progress through their sessions.

PART 1

- -

Understanding concentration

- -

We all know that in order to accomplish a certain thing we must concentrate.

It is of the utmost value to learn how to concentrate.

To make a success of anything you must be able to concentrate.

(Dumont, 2006, p15)

Concentration is like a well-honed blade.
When it gets blunt it needs sharpening.

(Bailey, 2012)

Concentration is like a well-honed blade.

Stigma and confusion about concentration

If improving concentration was easy, we would all have done it by now (Bailey & Brown, 2012). However, there has been, and continues to be, stigma and confusion over the concentration difficulties that a person experiences (Bailey & Brown, 2013). Some examples will help to capture the 'flavour' of the stigma and confusion arising from concentration difficulties.

Example 1 – the class with the 'class clown' who continually turns to chat to others. They do not listen to instructions, they fiddle with things, they daydream while others are on task. The teacher repeatedly requests a better focus from this individual yet seems to be ignored by them.

As a result, the teacher gradually becomes less tolerant of the individual who it appears cannot retain an instruction or ignores directives to be quiet and settle down to the task.

Example 2 – a person believes that their concentration 'weakness' is a neurological disorder and, as a result, they consider the concentration difficulty to be outside their control and something they cannot alter.

Believing in this, they fail to respond to the attempts of their educators, clinicians, teachers or parents to control them through command or criticism. They expect to be challenged or criticised and often feel helpless to respond. This is a difficult pattern to break and is likely to become a repeated and an embedded pattern of behaviour.

Example 3 – a teacher or parent is unimpressed by an individual's lack of response to instructions and their apparent lack of change to negative consequences. Their behaviour does not vary. As a result, a cycle begins where the teacher or parent can be increasingly frustrated by the individual's apparent lack of concern about the impact of their behaviour on both their own learning and that of others. The teacher or parent is left thinking, and continuing to think, the individual should 'know better' and be able to control themselves.

Example 4 – an adult employee is frequently making errors in assembling a product at work. They did well on the training course for the production line, coming out in the top 5 per cent. The excellent results were sent back to the work supervisor. The production line training course was run in 30-minute segments with 10-minute breaks between each course module. However, at work, this is not the case.

At work, the person has to work for 2 hours before their break time. Unfortunately, no one at work knows that the adult can only concentrate and perform well for about 40 minutes before they become confused, can't think straight and feel fatigued. Instead, the employee is berated for being lazy – a shirker – and is verbally abused by other employees, who refuse to work alongside them. The employee is at risk of losing their job.

Concentration lies at the heart of learning. Yet, until recently, little was known about exactly how to improve concentration (Brown & Bailey, 2013). However, by changing the way we think about and conceptualise concentration, we can find ways in which individuals can learn to better manage and improve their concentration (Bailey, 2012).

Are you concentrating?

Have you ever experienced a time when you were trying to settle to a task but you just could not? And, instead of getting on with the task, you had a minor lapse of concentration and engaged in task-irrelevant activities?

We all experience these minor lapses in concentration occasionally. We may be trying to listen to someone and take in what they are saying, yet interesting ideas 'pop' into our mind from nowhere and divert our attention from what is being said. This may be because our own thoughts are more interesting to us than the ideas of the person we are listening to. Or, it may be just because the ideas are there and any thoughts interrupt our focus.

> **Work** – Are you someone who can work better without interruptions or distractions? If so, how do you cope when the mobile phone keeps ringing or when other people interrupt your thinking?
>
> **Education** – Classroom environments can also be distracting. For example, some students are easily distracted by other people in their class. Even when we have a peaceful environment to work in, we might be torn between varying demands or desires, or find it hard to switch our attention from one task to another.

These types of challenge to concentration are common to most people. We need to stop and think about how we might improve our concentration. When we begin to think about our concentration skills and experiences, it soon becomes evident that we hardly ever think about them in detail. Yet we find many people are quite dismissive and often judge themselves in a negative way. For example, one student says 'I am useless at concentrating' and another, 'I can only concentrate when I am interested in something.'

In most people's minds there is a strong link between concentration and performance. But not many could explain how they went about concentrating, or what they might do to enhance their performance, if their concentration is poor. Often, people with concentration difficulties are repeatedly told to 'concentrate harder'. This implies that concentration is something that can be accomplished simply through applying willpower. The result: many students with concentration concerns are stigmatised at school and college with labels such as 'lazy', 'time-waster' or 'lacks discipline'. However, there is a real problem here. If we don't know what we have to do to concentrate, how can we be expected to improve?

Surprisingly, concentration need *not* be difficult to do. It can even be a highly pleasurable experience. It is something we can all do and it is something that everyone can learn how to do better.

This resource book aims to dispel some of the myths about concentration. It also provides a framework through which individuals can understand the mechanisms of concentration and begin to learn how to improve their own performance.

A little bit of history

Concentration and its importance in human performance grew out of theories and studies of stress, state-dependent learning, perception, attention, memory, and cognitive psychology (Best, 1955; Treisman, 1960, 1964; Lazarus, 1966; Neisser, 1967, 1976; Moray, 1969; Selye, 1976, 1979; Rossi, 1993).

Historically known as 'focalisation' (James, 1890), concentration concerns the allocation of mental activity (Kahneman, 1973). Against this historical background, we can see that concentration involves attentional, cognitive, environmental, behavioural and emotional states of mind (Brown & Bailey, 2011). We view 'concentration as a state of mind which reflects the ability of the individual to apply themselves to a task(s) without interference from distractions' (Bailey & Brown, 2012).

Concentration can be likened to an orchestra that is noisy and chaotic until it is tuned up. When it is, the brain, like the orchestra, enlists different functions or domains to act in concert with each other to enhance attention and concentration.

(Bailey & Brown, 2013, p3)

Sometimes called 'focused concentration' (Lezak *et al*, 2004), it is the capacity to attend to one or two events or ideas, while at the same time blocking out awareness of competing distractions.

Practically speaking, it is not possible or desirable to concentrate all of the time. What is important is to be able to concentrate when it is needed and appropriate. Unfortunately, we cannot always concentrate when we need to. We all at some point know what it is like to have a 'wandering mind' (Bailey & Brown, 2012; Brown & Bailey, 2013).

Some of the time when we are not concentrating as well as we should be, there are no harmful effects or serious consequences for us or other people. However, where there is a significant lack of focused concentration in education, work and sporting performance, or in our personal relationships, significant errors of judgement and decision making occur. During these 'failures of concentration episodes' (Bailey, 2012), we can perform and behave in ways that narrow or block our performance. Where this happens, it makes us and others vulnerable and can lead to undesirable outcomes. Some examples are listed below.

Examples of failures of concentration episodes

- A driver fails to stop and drives through a red traffic light.

- A student completes their homework but for the wrong assignment.

- A manager in a print works approves a book run which has many spelling errors.

- An accounts manager signs a cheque for goods that were never purchased.

- A ship's captain makes a navigational error and runs the ship onto rocks.

- A pupil in a lesson chats with friends and misses what the teacher says.

- Two people never agree because they only focus on their weaknesses.

- A student understands the assignment but 'forgets' it when writing it down.

- An athlete takes the wrong turn during a marathon race.

- A pilot overshoots a runway they use daily on a familiar flight path.

- The driver of a touring bus reads a map wrongly and drives into a ravine.

- A sales manager is so tired he signs an important contract he has not read.

- A student does not listen and fails to turn up for an important examination.

- A train passenger pulls the 'emergency stop' lever instead of the heater switch.

- A body shop paint manager misjudges the paint colour needed for a car.

- A professional snooker player misses easy shots and loses to a lesser player.

- A student takes too long to focus their attention and fails to complete tasks on time.

- A machine operator fails to check safety equipment and has a serious accident.

Capacity for concentration

One of the salient difficulties for children and adults who demonstrate performance problems at school and at work and in sports performance is their limited capacity for concentration. However, the capacity for concentration can vary between individuals and within the same person at different times under different conditions. Emotional stress factors such as anxiety, anger, depression and

 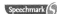

mental fatigue can all interfere with, and reduce the capacity for, concentration in children and adults (Bailey, 2010; Brown & Bailey, 2011). In particular, brain injury and developmental disorders may all reduce the capacity for concentration in both temporary and more permanent ways (Lezak *et al*, 2004). Some examples are listed below.

Examples of reduced capacity for concentration

- A recently bereaved person 'can't concentrate' on routine tasks

- An anxious adolescent blocks their capacity to concentrate.

- An angry child fails to focus on what they are doing.

- A tired student cannot organise their thoughts.

- A pupil takes on a task that is beyond their cognitive ability.

- A depressed employee can't concentrate for very long.

- A child whose parents are divorcing starts 'daydreaming'.

- A brain-injured victim of a road traffic accident can no longer focus.

- A student with attention deficits has a variable capacity to concentrate.

- A head-injured pilot can no longer concentrate on daily briefings.

- A business executive needs frequent breaks to focus on what he has to do.

Concentration span

People with concentration difficulties are sometimes said to have a 'poor concentration span'. Concentration span concerns how much information can be grasped at once and processed at any one time on a given task. However, children and adults who do have a poor concentration span may do so for many different reasons. These include emotional distress, psychological and physical trauma, trauma cognitive impairment, or through ageing (Brown & Bailey, 2011). Here, concentration span means *a state of mind which reflects the ability of the individual to apply themselves to a task **over time** without interference from distractions*. Being able to maintain and increase your concentration span on a task is crucial for achieving educational, relational, work and sports goals (Moran, 2004; Sadhu, 2004; Dumont, 2006; Griffey, 2010).

Divided and alternating concentration

Divided and alternating concentration involves the ability to focus on more than one task at a time or to focus on multiple elements within a complex cognitive or behavioural task. It can also entail moving between two or more tasks simultaneously. In particular, alternating concentration concerns placing demands on the person to shift their focus from one task to another and back again. Divided and alternating concentration can also be very fragile and sensitive to changes that reduce the capacity for memory and coding-retrieval of information by the individual (Craik *et al*, 1996). An example will highlight the vulnerabilities of divided and alternating concentration.

Example of divided and alternating concentration

A waiter approaches three diners in a restaurant, welcomes them and asks for their order. The diners order three glasses of lime and soda, two club sandwiches and a tuna panini. During the ordering, they get into conversation with the waiter about his home town and share their experiences about travel. In the middle of this conversation, they say they want to add a portion of French fries to the order. The desultory conversation continues for another few moments; the waiter recalls experiences he had before moving to his current job. He then leaves the diners and places their order.

When it is ready, he returns to their table with the drinks, club sandwiches and the panini. But no French fries. For the waiter, the order is complete. The diners notice there are no French fries accompanying their order and mention this to each other.

What happened here? Clearly, the waiter was distracted, his concentration was divided, and he had to alternate between concentrating on the small-talk conversation of the customers and the order they were making. It was a typical task for a waiter. One he completed but not without error. On another day and with other customers – even the same customers – the task would be carried out error-free.

This is a good example of what can happen – and does happen – when we have to divide and switch our concentration from one task to another and back again.

Impaired concentration

Taking these different aspects of concentration together, people with difficulties in attention and concentration are often characterised by slower processing abilities. Many of these impairments are among the most common in educational and mental health problems and in individuals with brain damage. It is a complex area. For instance, the individual's cognitive functions may be intact.

Speechmark

They may be cognitively capable, yet adversely affected through emotional stress and fatigue (Lezak *et al*, 2004). Clearly, emotional stress and fatigue in a person can result in impaired concentration (Bailey, 2012).

Concentration difficulties

Concentration difficulties can present significant problems for individuals in education, business and sport. The typical difficulties in concentration that people report are:

- My mind wanders.

- I can't think straight.

- I feel angry and agitated.

- I forget instructions.

- I rush tasks too much.

- I am easily distracted.

- I feel anxious and on edge.

- It's hard for me to prioritise.

- I feel tired.

- I find it hard to switch from one thing to another.

- I need regular breaks.

- I can't seem to get started on a task.

Concentration and ageing

Changes in brain activity that begin gradually in middle age may explain why older adults have a harder time concentrating in busy environments, and are easily distracted by irrelevant information. Comparing brain functions in young, middle-aged and older adults, Campbell *et al* (2012) found that older adults are more easily distracted than younger people.

These findings suggest that, in older adults, a *reduced functional connectivity* occurs within the frontoparietal network, manifesting in the frontal based control mechanisms of the brain. It appears that a *see-saw imbalance* affects the individual, swinging between blocking distraction and being easily distracted. Often starting in middle to later age (40–60 years), the see-saw pattern probably adversely breaks down in older adults, causing them to become less efficient at blocking distracting information than younger people. This see-saw imbalance probably becomes even more pronounced in older adults (aged 65+), which could explain why they seem to have a reduced ability to ignore distracting or irrelevant information (Campbell *et al*, 2012).

Subtle lapses in concentration

Clearly, not all of the concentration difficulties experienced by a person have costly consequences for them or what they are doing. Indeed, to the untutored eye, lapses in concentration may pass unnoticed. However, sometimes the consequences of even small lapses in concentration can be fatal, such as those injuries incurred by the victims of road traffic accidents. In such cases, impaired concentration can literally be bad for our health and survival. As well as having concerns over their health and safety, individuals with problems in concentrating risk undermining their relationships and educational, work and sports performance.

Some of the subtlest adverse effects on our cognitive ability and psychological functioning are those daily or episodic breaks in our concentration which, although not life-threatening, can threaten our learning. A typical example is the student who has lapses in concentration and 'fails to listen' to which pages need reading for a science project. This is sometimes wrongly attributed by teachers as 'forgetting homework', when it is a clear case of lapses in concentration.

The wandering mind

Many lapses in concentration occur because our mind wanders away from the task we are supposed to be concentrating on. But why does it wander? According to the eminent American psychologist William James (1842–1910), the 'wandering mind' wanders because of involuntary activity and interesting external events, that seize our attention (James, 1890; Moran, 2004). However, this does not explain why our mind wanders during sleep, when we are unaware of events in the external world (Moran, 2004). It also doesn't account for the mind wandering during creative activity (Bailey, 2012). We need to be clear that individuals are not thought of as having a wandering mind simply because they are 'weak-willed' or 'lack the willpower' to resist fascinating external events.

A radical approach to understanding the wandering mind is to consider it as purposeful – part of the 'architecture of the mind'. Within this framework, we view the wandering mind as reflecting 'design features' of the mind at work (Moran, 2004). When we do this, we see that the wandering mind, and lapses in concentration do not happen because of the whimsical nature of the will. Our mind wanders because it probably evolved to do so!

Also, it may seem paradoxical but *our mind wanders because we try to control it* (Wegner, 1994; Moran, 2004). For example, if you try not to think of a pink elephant, what happens? You probably created an image or a thought of a pink elephant before you were able not to think of it. It's a paradox of the mind: we *have* to think of something we *don't* want to think about before we can stop thinking about it. Trying to think about not staying awake when we want to get to sleep is another example. But why do we do it?

Speechmark

It is because of what Wegner (1994) called 'ironic' mental processing. There may be evolutionary reasons for engaging in ironic mental processing. It may give the mind a natural rest – a break from stress or fatigue – and ease the mental load involved in concentrating (Moran, 2004; Bailey, 2012).

Ironic mental processing may also act as an environment scanner. It allows us to check the environment for relevant or irrelevant events, or for potential harm or threats to our physical and psychological safety (Wegner, 1994; Bailey, 2013).

When we *are* able to apply our concentration and prevent our mind from wandering, we probably use a different set of mental processes. Wegner (1994) refers to these as part of an 'intentional' operating system which relies on intentional mental processes. In many tasks, we can rely on our intentional operating system to exercise more control over our mind than our ironic mental processing. However, as Moran (2004) observes, this can 'rebound' and we experience the thought we were trying suppress. There is also evidence that people who try concentrating while being distracted are inclined to memorise the distractors because they cannot ignore them (Zuckier & Hagen, 1978).

Wegner (1997) developed the theory of ironic processes of mental control which is relevant to concentration. This theory says that:

> *both the most and the least desired effects of attempts to control one's own mental states accrue from two processes – an intentional operating process (a conscious, effortful search for mental contents that will produce a desired state of mind) and an ironic monitoring process (an unconscious, automatic search for mental contents that signal a failure to produce the desired state of mind). Although the monitoring process usually functions just to activate the operating process, during stress, distraction, time urgency, or other mental load, the monitor's effects on [the] mind can supersede those of the operator, producing the very state of mind that is least desired. An individual's attempts to gain mental control may thus precipitate the unwanted mental states they were intended to remedy.*

> (Wegner, 1997, p148)

Adopting this perspective, we can appreciate why it can be difficult for people to control, direct and maintain their concentration. Knowing this, instead of vainly trying to control concentration through willpower, we can better direct our efforts at managing, regulating and 'taming' the wandering mind. This revelation should end useless and unhelpful attributions made about children and adults as having a wandering mind because they are weak-willed or have insufficient willpower. Clearly,

Speechmark

understanding the wandering mind has enormous implications for anyone engaged in working with people who have concentration difficulties and are affected by distraction.

Distraction – causes and effects

Distraction is defined on Wikipedia as 'the divided attention of an individual or group from the chosen object of attention onto the source of distraction'. Distraction is caused by:

- a lack of ability to pay attention

- a lack of interest in the object of attention

- the great intensity, novelty or attractiveness of something other than the object of attention.

Distractions can come from both external and internal sources. Viewed as a stimulus, distraction is seen as being out there – in the external environment. External distraction arises from distractors such as noise, heat, cold and light. Internal distractions come from within the person. These internal distractors can be intrusive images or thoughts, impulsive behaviour, boredom, stress, unwanted emotions, fatigue and perturbing body sensations such as pain. Here distraction is defined as *arising from the interaction between the person, their environment and the task they are carrying out* (Bailey & Brown, 2012).

Clearly, individuals can't concentrate all the time. Nor should they be expected to. Also, having appropriate breaks from concentration are often helpful for the individual to 'refresh 'and return their focus to tasks they are in the process of completing. Being aware of their concentration profile can assist individuals to reduce distractions and improve their 'concentration time' (Brown & Bailey, 2012).

Distraction management

One way of managing distraction is to help people identify their distractors, and to get better at evaluating and managing those external situations and internal states that distract them. Here this is called 'distraction management' (DM):

> *Distraction Management can be defined as the degree to which a person can ignore task irrelevant information over time.*

(Bailey, 2013)

Distraction management can be highly productive and profitable for individuals, their performance, and relationships with others and in reducing costs to organisations (Moran, 2004). Effective DM is something that we all need to learn. Yet DM does not seem to be taught in school, college, university, or in the world of work. We need to look to the psychology of concentration in sports to appreciate how important distraction management is for sports performers (Moran, 2004).

For many athletes, concentration training is now part of their preparation for competitive sporting events. A significant part of concentration training is to manage distractors. Simulation and behaviour rehearsal can be useful here. For example, as part of their preparation, a squad of athletes who need to perform next to a noisy railway station, before the event could find a park near a main-line station and carry out their training session exposed to the noise of trains. Equally, internal distraction – the 'noise' of the mind–body, intrusive thoughts, disruptive emotions and felt bodily pain, discomfort or fatigue – can *adversely* affect preparation for examinations, academic performance, driving safely, carrying out procedures, operating equipment, sporting achievement, and doing productive work.

Clearly, when people have significant erratic and unmanageable intrusive concentration difficulties, it can lead them to make costly human errors. These difficulties can be episodic, prolonged, wide-ranging and include errors of attribution, feeling, thinking, judgement and action. Where these difficulties persist, it is also essential to consider the role motivation may be playing in interfering with or impairing the person's concentration.

Motivation and concentration

Motivation is not concentration. Anybody working with an individual on concentration needs to be aware of the part that motivation can play in improving their concentration. For example, motivation can significantly influence an individual's ability to maintain good levels of focus on-task and to persist in their performance at points of difficulty. This is one good reason why it is useful for coaches and educators to consider the possible role of motivation in contributing to, or interfering with, an individual's ability to concentrate.

Motivation on-task can be affected by:

- the level of interest in the activity

- the nature of the task

- whether or not an individual feels competent in their ability to carry out the task efficiently.

Motivation is also affected by external factors such as task demands and the time set to complete a task. Where the tasks set are demand-led, it is useful to explore with the person:

1   the level of control they have over the task

2   how secure they feel about carrying out the task

3   what level of support they might require.

It is also worth noting that some students can have difficulty with open-ended, unstructured tasks. So they may need support to break down such tasks into subsidiary components, to make the task manageable in some way. There is a strong relationship between the perception of a task and an individual's motivation to focus on and attend to it. When discussing activities with students, they can often engage in tasks where their concentration can be extensive and sustained for lengthy periods. However, on other tasks, their ability to sustain focus and attention can be adversely affected. How the complexity of the task is perceived can also affect students' motivation to carry out a task (Perlmutter & Monty, 1977; Perlmutter & Chan, 1983). As a consequence of their perception, students' motivation can influence how and when they begin to engage on the task.

The authors believe that intrinsic motivation – that which personally energises and motivates the student – is fundamental to understanding and increasing motivation. Edward Deci's cognitive evaluation theory model of intrinsic motivation (Deci & Porac, 1978) closely aligns with the authors' views on motivation and its relationship to concentration.

Intrinsic motivation is what matters most to the student, and their thoughts and feelings of competence and control. *The student needs not only to control their task environment but also to think and feel competent in that control.* By overcoming challenging situations and tasks, the student begins to feel competent, and their motivation to engage in tasks is strengthened.

> *Intrinsic motivation generates behaviors that cause a person to feel competent and self-determining. These behaviors are of two kinds. First, if stimulation is low, intrinsic motivation will generate behavior to increase stimulation. Second, intrinsic motivation will lead to behavior involved with conquering challenges.*

(Petri, 1996, p331)

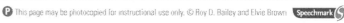

Exploring the intrinsic motivations of students is important because it allows each individual to access relevant personal information and decide how best to motivate themselves for a particular task. When this is done well, the student is enabled to identify and act on the relationship between their motivation and concentration. In doing so, the student may find that they do not have a problem with concentration directly but more of a problem with motivation on-task. Moreover, emotional stress can often be increased by setting tasks in which an individual has limited control but the demands are high (Bailey, 2010).

Empowering individuals to make informed choices and feel more resourceful and in control of tasks is likely to have a mediating impact on reducing stress levels (Perlmutter & Monty, 1977; Perlmutter & Chan, 1983; Glasser, 1985, 1990; Seligman, 2004; Bailey, 2012). Such arrangements can also encourage an individual to become calmer, more confident and goal-orientated, and to retain focused concentration, leading them to be more efficient on-task (Bailey & Brown, 2012).

Motivation and concentration are linked through the choices we make: about what we think, say, feel and do. These choices depend on the goals we want to aspire to and the behaviours that lead to us to our goals. Our goals are held in our heads as 'cognitive representations of some future state' – beliefs and expectations that behaviours we choose will lead us to a desired goal. This is what also motivates us to concentrate.

A typical example is a student wanting, believing and expecting to receive a university degree will be motivated to concentrate on their studies (Petri, 1996). This increases the likelihood that they will achieve their goal and feel good about themselves. Yet motivation can be variable. Not all students can maintain sufficient motivation to concentrate on their studies that they reach the 'finishing line'.

Clearly, just as motivation may vary, concentration does too. Looked at in this way, *concentration can also be understood as a particular state at any one time and over time. Concentration is therefore as much a process as a state*. It was this understanding that led the authors to develop the Concentration Assessment Profile* (CAP) system (Bailey & Brown, 2013).

Concentration as a process

The process model of concentration is also a coaching model and addresses the social and psychological domains associated with difficulties in concentration. The CAP and model (Bailey & Brown, 2013) provides the basis for evaluation and creating coaching intervention for people who have concentration difficulties.

The domains relating to concentration difficulties function within an internal and an external environment of facilitators and distractors which are significant for each person. The model covers five main domains of concentration difficulty (as overleaf). These difficulties in concentration are associated with:

* This is a professional resource for profiling and evaluating concentration difficulties against our process model of concentration. It is available from Speechmark Publishing, London.

1   receiving information

2   the thinking involved in it

3   carrying out actions which relate to concentration.

The model also takes into account:

4   emotional stress

5   environmental factors reported by each individual.

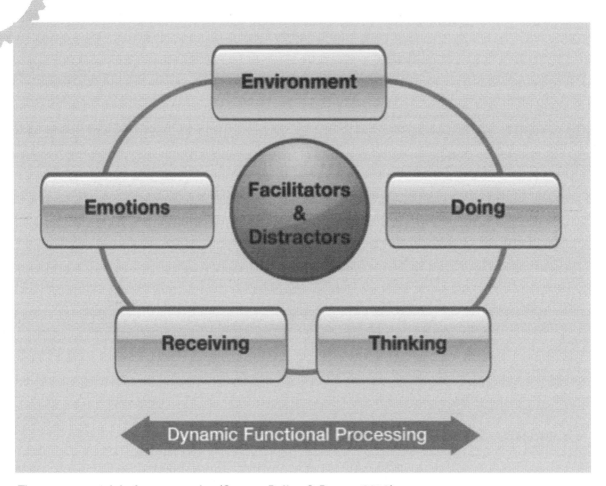

The process model of concentration (Source: Bailey & Brown, 2013)

Facilitators and distractors

Facilitators and distractors are relevant within each of the domains of concentration in the CAP model. Clearly, they can influence concentration. In the model:

- facilitators are those situations or conditions within each domain that may significantly contribute to promoting or maintaining concentration

- distractors are those situations or conditions within each domain that can interfere with and undermine concentration.

Distractors can prevent us from concentrating or interrupt our concentration and lead to underperformance and errors in sport performance, work and education. Distractors can be either internal, and produced by the person, or external to the individual.

There are two main types of distraction —internal and external. Internal distractions include the voice in your head (that constant, sniping, irritating, internal critic) and daydreaming, while external distractions include the telephone ringing, noises in the street, other people. There's no doubt that some people are more easily distracted than others, but it is also possible to learn how to filter out distraction – which is very worthwhile, because research has shown that those who are more easily distracted produce worse test results.

(Griffey, 2010, p64)

Some examples of facilitators and distractors are given below.

Concentration is facilitated when:

- the body is running efficiently within limits (eg regulated body temperature, heart rate, respiration)

- the person experiences balance, calmness and emotional control

- the person is motivated to do a task

- the person can be selective in their attention and filter out irrelevant information

- what we are doing does not interfere with receiving and thinking about a relevant task

- we engage in task-relevant thinking

- the task environment is not overly demanding

- the person wants to do the task.

Concentration is impaired when:

- the body is running inefficiently (eg because of a cold or flu or backache, etc)
- the person experiences intrusive stress (eg anxiety, frustration, boredom, anger)
- the person is not motivated to do a task
- we cannot be selective in our attention and filter out irrelevant information
- what we are doing interferes with receiving and thinking about a relevant task
- we engage in irrelevant thinking
- the task environment is overly demanding
- a task is meaningless to the person.

There are many kinds of facilitators and distractors. They can range from our state of mind and emotions at the time to different sounds and sights in our surroundings. Each person has their own facilitators and distractors. For example, one person may like playing music to help them concentrate. Another may find that music acts as a distractor, preventing them from concentrating or interrupting their concentration. One person's facilitator may be another's distractor.

Facilitators and distractors can be stable or vary over time. Therefore, it is also helpful to identify individual facilitators and distractors when assessing, evaluating and improving concentration. Why is this? Because it is useful in helping us choose and create the conditions whereby we can increase the presence of our facilitators and, at the same time, reduce or remove distractors that we find adversely affect concentration.

Processing information

Distraction can occur when we have to attend to, listen to, think about and process information. Individuals can quickly become overloaded with information and have memory and processing difficulties which might impact on their ability to focus in this mode. They may find that their mind wanders easily when having to receive information. It may have more to do with the type of information being delivered as to whether or not a student can concentrate on that information, or it might be universally applied across all modes of listening or receiving type activities.

Time factors might be important. Indeed, research suggests that people can only cope with up to 10 minutes' worth of information and that memory may be adversely affected accordingly. Yet individuals can vary in how well they can attend to something (Wilson & Koran, 2007). However, some people find it difficult to listen in an active mode. For others, combining sitting still with receiving information can be quite a difficult process. The environment might make a difference.

 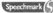

For example, if a student is relaxed and reading information personally, to take in information, they may find this process quite easy but, at other times, difficult.

Meaningful information

Typically, people are inclined to concentrate on information that is personally meaningful to them in some way (Bailey, 2001; Griffey, 2010). For example, a student who wants to do well – either for themselves or for their parents – is more likely to focus their concentration on the subject at school, and do meaningful homework assignments, than a student for whom a task has little or no meaningful information.

Information becomes meaningful to us when we appraise and evaluate it as having personal significance for us. The personal significance of information can act as a motivator or an inhibitor to our concentration. It can also help us to cope with task demands or lead to unwanted stress (Bailey & Clarke, 1989).

> *When it comes to concentrating on something, it's much easier if the task has meaning for you and is something you can engage with. Often concentration becomes easier once you have been concentrating for a while, because what it is you are concentrating on starts to have greater meaning for you, the longer you concentrate on it. Even watching a movie requires you to watch for long enough to engage with its contents. Reading a book is the same. It's unusual to engage fully with the first few pages – people talk about 'getting into a book' or a book being 'difficult to get into' – but ... if you continue reading long enough, the brain engages with the content and concentration becomes easier.*

(Griffey, 2010, p111)

With meaningless or irrelevant information, the individual can often be unmotivated and have little interest in preparing for or concentrating on the task at hand. Another way of understanding this relationship to concentration is to view meaningful information as being 'hot' information and non-meaningful information as 'cold' information (Bailey, 2001).

- Hot information is directly or indirectly significant to the individual. Good examples are a homework assignment, a work project, or preparation for participation in a sporting event.

- Cold information has no personal meaning for the person. Good examples are numbers on a scale, how many grains of sand in a desert, or how often waves crash on the shore.

Thinking

Thinking involves being able to structure and organise information, consider factors and make sense of the information delivered. Thinking means being able to engage in a degree of introspective reflection. Some people can find it very hard to separate out thinking and doing. They have a tendency to fuse both factors together. Others find it very difficult to visualise, structure and organise information in their mind. They may require external assistance to engage in productive thought processes.

Other people can be so 'lost' in the thinking process, their minds 'drift off' in a diffuse, creative, expansive fashion. Some internally focused individuals can be so overly ponderous in their thinking that they have difficulty in completing tasks. Another drawback of 'over-inclusive thinking' is that it can create too much mind 'noise' and inhibit decisiveness and actions.

'Straight' and 'crooked thinking' (Thouless, 1971) can help or hinder our concentration and performance on tasks that require clear analytical and logical thought. Inappropriate thinking can also contribute to impaired concentration. It is an area that a coach may find evident in some students. In this case, the coach's task is to empower the student in such a way that they identify what their thinking difficulty is, its source and how this impairs their concentration. Each case is different, but the coach should also keep in mind that a student's inappropriate thinking may be linked to learning difficulties. Thinking needs to be recognised as a specific area of cognitive processing which can facilitate or adversely affect the individual's focus and attention.

Environmental factors also need to be considered for their influence on thinking. Questions such as where and what environments help increase or reduce the individual's awareness of their difficulties with thinking need to be closely investigated. A better understanding of the relationship between 'learning' environments and distracted or inappropriate thinking can help us to manage and reduce obstacles to concentration.

Emotional stress

There is a direct relationship between emotional stress and impairments in concentration (Bailey, 2010). When an individual becomes preoccupied by emotional stress, this can have an adverse effect on their ability to focus their attention across a broad spectrum of different task-type issues. If the individual has any deep-seated anxieties, this can also upset their sense of calmness to the point where they cannot listen, think clearly and 'settle down' to activities.

Emotional stress can also disrupt concentration in other ways. An individual can begin a task well but then find that their mind is constantly interrupted by intrusive thoughts. These thoughts may be driven by anxiety, which is a clear indicator of emotional stress. Where achievement is important, emotional stress can lead to intrusive thoughts and self-doubt about being able to do or complete a task. Clearly, intrusive thinking can undermine focused attention.

Emotional stress and related factors can be resolved and better managed through assisted self-evaluation by a performance facilitator or coach. It is often relevant to explore with an individual the nature of their feelings about particular activities they are engaged in and how this impinges on their ability to retain good levels of focus. It is also important to elicit the self-talk which emerges as an individual is progressing through a task which requires sustained, focused concentration. Looking at their self-talk, we can examine in detail whether its content is cyclical and if it generally undermines or assists their performance.

Students who have difficulties concentrating within a group environment can be affected by emotional stress. This often arises from a fear of failure or concerns about being 'shown up' in some way within the group environment. Some students with learning difficulties cope with emotional stress by adopting a task-avoidance strategy. This may be their 'best' attempt to avoid embarrassment or being ridiculed by their peer group and concerns about their performance.

Some patterns of behaviour suggest that students can experience emotional stress and agitation as a result of feeling under threat from the classroom environment. Some patterns formed in early childhood are difficult for the child to break. In such instances, the child can become unhelpfully labelled as a student with 'poor' concentration when, in fact, the 'poor' concentration may have grown out of emotional trauma they experienced earlier in their childhood. When we are emotionally charged or distressed, it can become difficult to focus and pay attention. This is particularly relevant when we are faced with new or unfamiliar tasks. It is easier to cope with tasks that are familiar and less personally demanding when feeling distressed or upset in any way.

Specific feelings can adversely affect concentration. Frustration is one. When engaged in an activity, if we begin to feel frustrated with the task, working through that frustration can be a particular skill requirement. Students who are already overloaded with emotional stress can find feelings of frustration so overwhelming that it becomes difficult to retain a good level of focus and application in their work.

Learning to deal with personal frustration is central to improving our concentration and task performance (Bailey, 2010). Students need to work through these issues and learn not to fight feelings of frustration. One way of doing this is to:

1 recognise feelings of frustration

2 become aware of changes within their body

3 acknowledge emotional stress

4 re-label frustrating thoughts as indicators that it is 'time to rethink'

5 return to the task when frustration has eased.

These and anger-management techniques can all prove useful in positively dissipating the frustration associated with emotional stress (Bailey, 2010).

Environmental factors

Where and when work is demanded of an individual plays a part in levels of focus and attention on task. Some people find it easier to work on tasks away from others and need quiet and orderly environments to be able to focus and attend. Others prefer visual stimulation or a noisy, busy environment. Working in a familiar, cosy atmosphere can facilitate concentration. Some individuals have set routines which they need to run through in order to focus their mind. Others can concentrate more easily on demand.

The time of the day can affect our concentration. Some people view themselves as 'early birds' who work best in the mornings. Others struggle to get up in the morning and prefer to put in work that requires good focus at the end of a day. These factors can affect people's ability to concentrate on demand within a 9-to-5 work environment or a school setting.

One of the main environmental factors that influence concentration is the requirement to perform within a group situation. This is the kind of environment where students report the greatest impact from distraction. The presence of other people in a room, particularly in a classroom, can have a detrimental impact on concentration. The reasons why other people being around has a negative impact on concentration abilities are many and varied. They need to be evaluated on an individual level, through discussion with the student concerned, if the environment is highlighted by the profile as being a key area causing concentration difficulties.

Working alone in a room can still cause problems for some people. There are those who find isolation unnerving, particularly if others elsewhere in a building are not engaged in work tasks. Interruptions to concentration can also impact on our ability to re-engage on a task. People who are trying to complete difficult tasks can find that mobile phone calls, social interruptions or even extraneous noises severely interfere with the flow of thinking necessary to complete tasks efficiently.

Doing tasks

Clearly, there are many individuals who can take in information well and have no difficulty with thinking about a task to be done, organising information, planning and structuring. However, the difficulty for them comes when the task actually needs to be carried out. For many, it is at this particular point that their actions begin to be affected by distractions. The 'doing' component of a task typically requires endurance, sustained motivation, an appropriate sense of time and time management, and an ability to keep going in the face of difficulty. The 'doing' phase may reflect a particular type of task where concentration is easily lost.

An individual may find that they can progress through an activity if it is a practical task, whereas with something which is more academic in its requirements it may be harder for them to sustain their

 Speechmark

efforts over time. Environmental factors can be significant in other ways. For example, some students find it particularly difficult to carry out a task within a group environment. For others, it is harder when they are alone and need to be self-motivated on-task.

One of the most common concentration difficulties people report is not having enough time to do or complete a task. Here there may be:

(a) specific issues about appreciating and managing time

(b) an inappropriate appraisal of the passage of time

or

(c) the student may become easily frustrated by limitations in their own competence or productivity during the time available to complete a task.

Attribution – making up our world

We all have to make sense of the world around us and give it meaning. We do this through how we receive information through our senses – what we think, feel and do about our experiences. We create and make up our mental world (Frith, 2007). By doing this, we engage in making up and explaining the world to ourselves and our attempts to understand other people (Bailey, 2012). Attribution is central to the way we go about discovering causes and effects (Kelly, 1967). Like intuitive scientists, we make attributions about ourselves, our interpersonal relationships and the world around us (Heider, 1958).

Creating attributions reflects our attempts to explain and understand why something causes something else, why someone has a particular gift or difficulty and why it occurs. Making valid attributions helps us in discovering knowledge about ourselves, other people and the situations we face in our lives. However, many of the attributions we make about ourselves, other people and situations are invalid. We simply get it wrong. These times can create problems – and they arise through errors of attribution.

Errors of attribution

Clearly, when considering concentration difficulties, it is important to avoid making errors of attribution. When we explain the reasons and causes for our behaviour, we can be inclined to adopt several cognitive biases and errors. For example, our perception of events can be distorted by:

- our past experiences
- our expectations
- our needs.

The most common types of misattribution include: interpersonal misattribution, predictive misattribution, explanatory misattribution, self-serving bias and fundamental attribution error. These are described in turn below.

Interpersonal misattribution

This happens when, for example, telling a story to a group of friends or acquaintances, we are inclined to tell it in a way which puts us in the best possible light. So, for instance, if you were telling a story about a waiter you fell out with in a restaurant, you would describe him as being aggressive, inattentive and rude and emphasise your patience and consideration.

Predictive misattribution

This is when we tend to misattribute things in a way which allows us to make future predictions, even though this may be invalid. For example, if your car was vandalised, you might misattribute the crime to the fact that you had parked in a particular part of a town. On this basis, you would avoid parking there in future, assuming you would avoid further vandalism to your car.

Explanatory misattribution

This is used to make sense of the world around us. Some people have an optimistic style of explanatory misattribution, while others tend to be more pessimistic. People with an optimistic style attribute positive events to stable, internal and global causes and negative events to unstable, external and specific causes. Those with a pessimistic style attribute negative events to internal, stable and global causes and positive events to external, stable and specific causes.

Self-serving bias

This is where we attribute success to internal factors. For example, if you did well in a test or an exam, the chances are you would say I did this well because I am smart or have the ability, or I did well because I studied and prepared well. Conversely, if you did badly, you are likely to attribute this to external forces. For example, you may say that you failed the test because the teacher included surprise questions, or the classroom was so cold you couldn't concentrate.

Note that self-serving bias is an attribution that leads to success being attributed internally and failure based on outside forces, rather than accepting personal responsibility.

Fundamental attribution errors

This is most vividly demonstrated when it comes to other people. Then we tend to attribute causes to internal factors, such as personality characteristics, and ignore or minimise external circumstances. This is what psychologists call fundamental attribution error. Even though situational variables are probably present, we automatically attribute causes to internal characteristics. For instance, when a person demonstrates concentration difficulties, we must take care to avoid the fundamental attribution error of automatically concluding it is because they are lazy or do not want to do the task. Social psychologists refer to this as 'blaming the victim' (Goldinger *et al*, 2003). For example, blaming the victim occurs when we blame innocent victims of crime for their own misfortune. This is a typical example of making a fundamental attribution error.

Avoiding the dangers of misattribution

The challenge is to avoid making errors of attribution. In understanding concentration and improving it, we have to decide which of the many possible causes legitimately accounts for a person's concentration difficulties. Inferring the causes of behaviour has long been one of the central concerns in psychology and in psychological assessment (Heider, 1958; Kelly, 1967).

Through a process of critical evaluation, using the concentration assessment profiling (CAP) system (Bailey & Brown, 2013), we can usefully contribute to the investigation of concentration difficulties. The authors believe the concentration tools described in this resource book and the domain process model of concentration can help in drawing valid inferences about why a person evidences concentration difficulties.

However, practitioners need to be critical and careful in their attributions about why a person has concentration difficulties. The critical evaluation of a person's concentration profile (Bailey & Brown, 2013) helps us to counteract misattributions about individuals, such as 'Lee never concentrates, he's just lazy' or 'Sophie never applies herself, she is unmotivated' or 'Stephen can never improve his concentration because he has ADHD' or 'Tan can't make any better track-training times, she refuses to focus on my programme'.

One of the main aims of assessing concentration is to identify with the individual concerned the factors that they consider are having an adverse impact on their levels of concentration (Brown & Bailey, 2012). The concentration assessment profile system (Bailey & Brown, 2013) provides this kind of information. It helps us to pursue an investigative process with the individual which can lead to them improving their concentration. It requires the individual concerned to have some ownership of the process. Through this they can increase their self-awareness and begin to seek out new ways to think about themselves in relation to concentration and their performance. With appropriate coaching and support, individuals and teams can learn new ways of improving their concentration.

Bringing it all together – domain equilibrium

When all of the domains of concentration are in balance, we call this domain equilibrium. It is a dynamic process and may change from stable to unstable equilibrium. Domain equilibrium can be high or low. Low domain equilibrium is vulnerable to imbalance and can be easily affected by distractors.

Distraction management is central to understanding and improving concentration. The better we can become at identifying and managing our facilitators and distractors, the more we can focus and maintain our level of concentration. However, the more significance or value distractors have for an individual, the more likely there is to be disruption and disequilibrium in their domains of concentration. Also, the greater instability in the domains of concentration, the more invasive distractors can be, adversely affecting concentration. An important goal in maintaining and improving concentration is to manage distractors. Effectively managing facilitators and distractors helps us to keep the process of concentration in balance.

The knowledge base and the model of concentration described here provide a platform for a better understanding of concentration. From here, working in partnership with individuals, they can be empowered to take practical steps to begin improving their concentration.

PART 2

Pathways to improving concentration

The longest journey begins with a first step.

(Lao-Tzu, 604–531 BC)

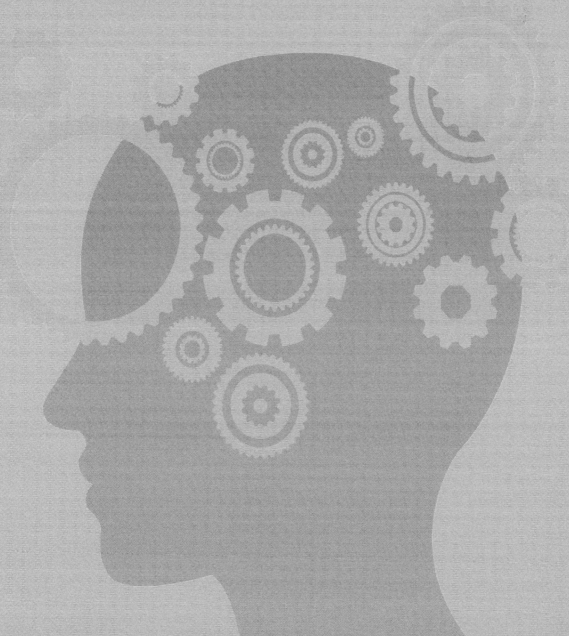

Introduction

There are several ways of improving concentration. Here, three main approaches are suggested:

1   Assessing and understanding concentration through profiling, using our assessment tool and process model of concentration

2   Learning within a mindful coaching framework to identify, evaluate and develop motivation and concentration skills

3   Practising concentration skills based on activities for improving concentration. These can be used either independently or linked to the process model of concentration, and assisted through coaching.

Using the domain process model of concentration

The process model of concentration can be used in the following ways, which are described further below.

- As a guide to understanding concentration.

- As a baseline before interventions to improve concentration.

- As a framework to consider concentration difficulties.

- As a platform for evaluating interventions.

- As an awareness-raising device.

A guide to understanding concentration

Using the domain process model of concentration, you can identify the main domains and distractors that undermine concentration. It can also be used to look at concentration at any moment in time, and over time. In this way, the model can give a 'snapshot' in time and a 'movie' of a person's concentration difficulties over a period of time. The model has also been designed to be used along with our Concentration Assessment Profile system (CAP) (Bailey & Brown, 2013). The CAP is used for assessing concentration difficulties and the severity of concentration problems in children and adults.

Importantly, because the model of concentration is a process model, it can be applied to understand how concentration difficulties may change over time and in different situations. For instance, one person may have more concentration problems in the morning than in the afternoon. Another person may have more problems in the afternoon than in the morning. More subtly, the same person may have both but alternating in some way.

The same considerations can also be applied to factors that facilitate concentration, as these may vary with time, situation and source. The process model of concentration helps you to see that one person's distractor can be another's facilitator and vice versa. More than this, it shows that, for the individual, their profile of concentration difficulties, although sometimes complex, can be understood.

A baseline before interventions to improve concentration

Having an understanding of concentration difficulties, the process model provides a baseline of where the person is at the time they are assessed. Using the process model of concentration and CAP in this way presents the coach, the educator and the clinician with a baseline profile of concentration difficulties. From such baselines, working with the person, you can design interventions and select activities to support their choices in improving their concentration.

Using the process model of concentration in conjunction with the CAP system (Bailey & Brown, 2013), you can easily and rapidly carry out multiple baseline assessments. This allows you to appreciate the similarities, differences and variations in a person's concentration difficulties. For example, you can tell when concentration is at its worst or least troublesome. Carrying out concentration difficulties baselines and multiple baselines, and interpreting them against the model, can map the 'character' of a person's concentration over time and their response to interventions to improve their concentration.

A framework to consider concentration difficulties

The process model of concentration also provides a clear framework within which to consider concentration difficulties. The attractiveness of such a framework helps to identify, analyse and formulate concentration difficulties in a way which can be understood by the person, the coach, the educator, the clinician, parents and others.

A key feature of the process model is that it can be used as a framework for appraising and evaluating concentration problems. This is something that we would also encourage the person to learn and apply. In the authors' experience, a working knowledge of the process model of concentration assists individuals in raising their awareness and self-evaluation of their concentration difficulties.

A platform for evaluating interventions

The process model of concentration can also be used to evaluate the effectiveness of specific activities for improving concentration. For example, a baseline assessment can be carried out with the individual and a profile of their concentration difficulties mapped. This can be done solely using the model to guide the analysis or in conjunction with the CAP (Bailey & Brown, 2013).

Working from the domains of concentration – receiving, thinking, feeling, doing, emotions and environment – you can analyse and identify which specific difficulties are more prevalent than others and how much they interfere with the individual's concentration. Information of this kind enables the coach to collaborate with the individual in selecting particular activities for improving concentration, and how they will be put into practice and reviewed or evaluated for their efficiency and effectiveness.

An awareness-raising device

Using the process model of concentration as an assessment device can be especially useful in raising the awareness of the person who is experiencing concentration difficulties (De Mello, 1997). To begin the process of self-awareness, the person needs to understand the nature of concentration and the way it relates to their own circumstances. It is as important to identify times when the person concentrates well as those when they have difficulties. This is because it is helpful feedback for the person to realise that their concentration difficulty is not necessarily all-encompassing and there could be many situations in which they concentrate perfectly well.

By helping the person to identify the distractors and facilitators in their concentration profile (Bailey & Brown, 2013), they can become more mindful of how well they are doing in the five domains of concentration – receiving, thinking, doing, emotions and environment. Mindful coaching is central to this process.

Mindfulness and mindful coaching

Mindful coaching empowers the person to better understand and improve their concentration. Mindful coaching can be effectively delivered through the conduit of mindfulness. There are different meanings and views about what mindfulness is (Gunaratana, 2002).

Some of these definitions are closely linked with meditation and see mindfulness as 'sati' or pure mind. Others relate more to understanding and improving concentration and mindful coaching (Bailey, 2012). The definition of mindfulness the authors believe relates well to mindful coaching is the one by John Kabat-Zinn (2003).

Mindfulness is:

> The *awareness* that *emerges* through *paying attention on purpose, in the moment,* and *non-judgementally* to the *unfolding of experience moment by moment*

> (Kabat-Zinn, 2003, emphasis added)

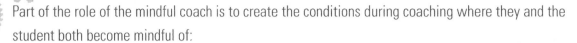

Part of the role of the mindful coach is to create the conditions during coaching where they and the student both become mindful of:

- emergent awareness
- paying attention on purpose
- in-the-moment awareness
- moment-by-moment awareness
- being non-judgemental
- unfolding of experience.

The authors have found four further psychological aspects that contribute to effective mindful coaching and can facilitate change:

- curiosity

- openness

- patience

- reflective thinking.

Accordingly, we conceive mindful coaching as follows.

> **Assisting the individual to create and cultivate new choices through an attitude of curiosity, openness, patience, in-the-moment and moment-by-moment awareness of information, reflective thinking, and to recognise non-judgementally the nature of their unfolding experiencing.**

Adopting this approach to mindful coaching, individuals can be empowered to recognise the concentration difficulties they may experience and how they could be overcome. This framework also helps us to get away from fallacious thinking such as invalid circular reasoning which assumes that a person's 'failure to concentrate' is the cause of their … *failure to concentrate*!

Through mindful coaching and using the model of concentration a person will realise that their so-called 'difficulties' arise from identifiable processes and sources which can be challenged and changed. For example, one student with low self-esteem, and labelled as being 'unable to concentrate', discovered that *they could concentrate* but could not carry out tasks in a noisy environment.

Coaching individuals to mindfully appraise and reflect on the factors and processes affecting their concentration, the mindful coach aims to empower people to better understand, manage and tame their 'wandering mind'.

A by-product of this process often empowers individuals to give up their negative view of themselves and develop a sense of positive wellbeing. This sense of wellbeing can help them to sustain their motivation when carrying out work, educational and sporting tasks in sometimes challenging environments.

Mindful coaching and the challenge of change

Not everything we face can be changed, but nothing can be changed unless we face it.

(Bailey, 1995)

When someone is struggling with a concentration problem, they can get stuck and believe they cannot change their situation, thinking, feelings, behaviour and emotional stress. In mindful coaching with individuals, we call this 'the challenge of change'. The challenge of change can appear daunting even when the individual wants to change, has insight into the nature of their behaviour, and has the ability to respond appropriately.

For example, it is not uncommon for some individuals to find it difficult to comply with guidance, even when their shortcomings are pointed out to them. This can be very frustrating. Why is it that some individuals don't do what is required of them? Life would be so much easier for them if they would just follow 'good' advice.

Many people with concentration difficulties are aware that they have 'a problem'. Yet consistently, they seem unable to change their view of themselves, their behaviour, thinking, feelings, emotional stress or situation. Apparently, they cannot find alternative ways of dealing with the difficulties they face. Clearly, it can be difficult to change thinking, feelings and behaviours that interfere with concentration, particularly if they are habitual. However, with mindful coaching, individuals become mindful and identify, evaluate, and make changes to their behaviour. Where mindful coaching, encouragement and challenge are sustained over time, individuals can and do adopt new choices, which improves their concentration.

We suggest that mindful coaching is a useful approach for working with individuals who want to change but may struggle to improve their concentration. We believe that a mindful coaching perspective provides a productive and useful form of support and challenge that is most likely to create the momentum for change in the individual concerned. However, to increase the likelihood of the individual making real progress in improving their concentration, much depends on the qualities and communication style of the coach.

The mindful coach and the individual

The authors' experience, and that of distinguished coaches, suggests that the qualities needed by a mindful coach are:

- observational skills

- empathy

- integrity

- openness

- a willingness to be flexible and responsive.

The communication style of the mindful coach is one of empowering the person to grow in confidence and competence.

Against this background, the mindful coach forms a 'working alliance' with the individual. The coach also facilitates the individual to become aware of, and take responsibility for, their choices and self-motivation. These come from within the individual and cannot be imposed externally. The individual's role is to find their 'treasures' – their psychological resources hidden in the mine of their mind. The coach's role is to work the mine with the individual.

Mindful coaching for improving concentration

Just as there are many pathways to improving concentration, there are also many different mindful coaching models to help a person improve their concentration and performance. For example, the GROW model of John Whitmore (2009) is used to enhance performance. Here, the coach assists the individual in identifying and specifying **G**oals, clarifying their current **R**eality, considering their **O**ptions, and harnessing their **W**ill and motivation to succeed.

In the mindful coaching model of concentration used here, for it to work well with the individual, the coach needs to emphasise:

- establishing rapport and trust

- facilitating personal learning

- sharing expectations and obtaining commitment

- prizing the person

- mindful coaching awareness

- empowering agreed performance

- individual awareness and personal responsibility

- asking questions and advancing understanding

- reviewing and evaluation

- concentration skills development.

Overview

Rapport and trust is the cement that holds the individual and coach together through the mindful coaching journey. It is the core of the mindful coaching relationship. It is a place where the individual can share their expectations and commitment with the coach, become more aware, and progressively take responsibility for their own learning and skills acquisition.

Evaluation is central to the mindful coaching model used here and takes into account the emergence of goals, choices and options of each individual. Advancing understanding is a key part of this model and addresses the reality and comprehension of concentration and how to improve it, by the individual.

Awareness is also recognised by Whitmore (2009) as central to mindful coaching and gaining control over performance.

The essential need is for each individual to be aware. Because we are only able to control what we are aware of, what we are unaware of controls us.

(Whitmore, 2009)

Against this background, we now take a closer look at our approach to mindful coaching and its relevance for improving concentration.

Establishing rapport and trust – the foundation

Establishing rapport and trust with the individual is the foundation on which their motivation will either grow and flourish or flounder and die. Without building and establishing rapport and trust with the individual, the coach is unlikely to be able to assist them in wanting to become aware of and better understand their concentration difficulties or how their concentration can be improved.

Another problem for the coach is that if they try to skip building and establishing rapport and trust with the individual, the individual may simply refuse to attend any mindful coaching sessions to help improve their concentration. This is a clear sign that the individual is not motivated to better understand or improve their concentration because they do not feel a rapport with the coach and do not have a shared foundation of trust.

Perhaps the greatest risk for the individual is when a coach fails to build and establish rapport and trust with the individual. In these circumstances, the individual may not be motivated to evaluate their learning or learn skills to improve their concentration. Clearly, establishing rapport and trust with the individual is essential to 'bringing out the best' in them. This can be greatly assisted by creating a mindful coaching climate with the individual in which they feel a sense of physical safety and emotional security.

Rapport and trust is the bread of communication (Bailey, 2001). This is why it is so important in mindful coaching to ensure that rapport and trust are built, established and continually nurtured between the coach and the individual. When rapport and trust are present, a synchronicity of behaviour is reflected between the coach and the individual. The coach needs to take steps to be competent in the skills of building rapport and trust with the individual, so as to engage in the process of mindful coaching.

Without rapport and trust, the coach runs the risk of creating a climate of fear for the individual. In such circumstances, the individual is unlikely to feel safe and secure or take any risks, such as identifying their concentration difficulties or committing to how they might improve their concentration.

Facilitating personal learning

Coaches also need to know how to facilitate the personal learning of individuals, that is, the kind of learning that will be relevant and meaningful to each individual. How can coaches begin to make this happen? What road is likely to lead to this progress and the satisfaction of individuals in education, sport and mindful coaching at work? The answer lies in the coach creating a facilitative learning climate with the individual.

In his seminal book *Freedom to Learn*, Carl Rogers (1969) identified the essential elements on which facilitative learning can be created and built. He found that facilitating personal learning has a significant impact on how we change, what we do, and what we learn.

How far along the road to facilitative learning are you as a coach? When you are working with an individual on their concentration and performance, you should:

- Communicate warmth and positive regard.

- Demonstrate genuineness to the individual.

- Communicate that you are open to and welcome their views, thoughts, feelings and behaviour.

- Listen carefully and accurately.

- Provide the individual with clear and rewarding feedback.

- Share bad news in a way in which constructive action can be taken.

- Communicate in ways that reflect your own thoughts, feelings and behaviour.

- Think, say, feel and do what you mean.

- Become individual-centred rather than coach-centred.

- Be genuine in your personal interactions with the individual.

Sharing expectations and obtaining personal commitment

Trust and rapport, although necessary to the coach–individual relationship, is not enough to empower the individual. It is here that the coach and individual relationship can falter and lose its direction for change. Quite simply, the coach and the individual need to achieve a clear definition of the performance expectations they should have of each other. Without it, how can a coach or an individual know how well they are doing? The problem is how you go about defining the expectations and who defines the performance that is required to improve the individual's concentration.

Clearly, what is expected between coach and individual should be made explicit, specific, achievable and measurable if possible. By doing this, you further reduce the risk of getting things badly wrong. Cutting down on the *expectation errors* now will go a long way to reducing problems the coach and individual may have to face in the future. This can be managed by the coach and individual being clear from the start what is expected from their performance. By making sure you get agreed performance right from the start, you will avoid having to make unnecessary changes of direction in the future.

Unless you agree with the individual and share your expectations of each other, a few problems can arise. First, you won't know where you are going. Second, you might think you agree when, in fact, there are different views of what should be done and how to do it. In this situation you will create a confusing communication cocktail for misunderstanding each other. A further difficulty is that you may fail to obtain the individual's personal commitment.

Unless the coach and the individual share and agree on expectations and reduce uncertainty to an acceptable level, they cannot achieve commitment. Yet the number of times when coaches and individuals fail to thoroughly discuss and agree on expectations is conspicuous by its absence. Sharing and agreeing performance expectations of each other is a necessary condition but often not sufficient for the individual to engage in real work with the coach to improve their concentration. Engagement with the coach requires the individual to make a personal commitment to working with the coach and on themselves.

To achieve personal commitment from the individual is *not* something you do as a coach. This may sound surprising – but personal commitment has to come from the individual. You cannot extract commitment from the individual as if you were squeezing juice from a lemon. It is the individual's decision to 'own' the performance expected from them that gives you the knowledge they will do their utmost to achieve the goals they set with you. Simply imposing the performances and goals we expect from an individual at best only gets compliance motivation, and compliance is a poor second to intrinsic motivation and personal commitment (Deci, 1975).

You run the risk of setting up unreliable and variable commitment when you decide and set the performances that are required by an individual without involving them throughout the process. Personal commitment comes from the individual participating with you in deciding, setting and evolving the performances required to achieve mutually desirable goals (Bailey, 2012).

Prizing the individual

When you create and communicate these conditions, you stop being self-centred. You start prizing the individual and not simply their performance. Prizing the individual occurs by conveying to them that they are worthy. Prizing the individual communicates the message 'I respect your contribution'. Above all, prizing the person enables them to believe in themselves (Rogers, 1986; Bailey, 1995).

Prizing the person is not a soft option. It sometimes means compassionately confronting them on aspects of their sabotaging behaviour, treasured beliefs, rigid thinking and strong feelings. However, this needs to be done in a way which gets the best out of the situation and still conveys positive regard for their views and their feelings. Prizing the individual is not directionless or without purpose. Prizing the person is not 'steam-rolling' them into doing what you want them to do. The aim of prizing the individual is to empower them to become aware of what is blocking their concentration and affecting their performance.

When you prize the individual, you provide opportunities for them to increase their awareness and discover their freedom to learn. When individuals themselves become more mindful, they discover their freedom to experience new learning. They are released from their limiting beliefs and inhibitions, their fears and defences.

Mindful coaching – how to survive in the snake pit

There is a scene in the film *Raiders of the Lost Ark* (1981) where Indiana Jones gets caught in a snake pit. Through sharpened awareness, great presence of mind and heroic composure, he survives and lives to pursue his next adventure. Empowering the individual through mindful coaching can be like that. Mindful coaching is exciting, but it can also be like walking through a snake pit. As a mindful coach, *you've got to watch where you place your feet* (Bailey, 1995). There are certain steps to take and others you need to avoid.

Steps to avoid

- Avoid treating concentration mindful coaching as an opportunity to boss or order people around.

- Avoid approaching concentration mindful coaching as an opportunity to manipulate individuals or groups simply to meet your own needs.

- Avoid pretending to engage in concentration mindful coaching when you have a secret agenda or devious intentions.

- Avoid using concentration mindful coaching as a means to off load and avoid your own responsibilities and goals.

- Avoid treating concentration mindful coaching as an excuse for inaction.

- Avoid practising concentration mindful coaching as if it is a soft option and does not involve careful thought, feelings and actions.

When you can avoid these dangers, you will have gone a long way towards combating mistakes in concentration mindful coaching. But you can go further than this: you can strengthen your approach to mindful coaching by making sure that you take the following steps.

Steps to take

- Convey respect, genuineness and positive regard during mindful coaching.

- Attempt to understand personal, educational, sporting or work issues as the individual sees them.

- Collaborate with the individual to make sense of their concerns, find appropriate solutions and take agreed action.

- Appreciate the values and motives that are linked to the individual's educational, sporting, occupational and personal priorities.

- Understand that mindful coaching is a process with the individual which takes time, and the outcomes are aimed at reaching agreed goals.

- Focus on where individuals are now and use this as a bridge to explore routes and paths to the future.

- Mobilise the present and, as yet, untapped personal resources of the individual so they can be aligned to achieve their future outcomes and goals.

- Expect the benefits of concentration mindful coaching to take effect – but remember, 'Rome wasn't built in a day'.

- Be patient! Individuals may need time to build new habits and refreshing repertoires that can lead to improving their concentration in education, sport and work.

Applying agreed performance

Having gone to the trouble of defining and sharing expectations and gaining commitment, the individual somehow has to apply the behaviour they have agreed with their coach. They have to find a way forwards – one that makes it possible for them to actually carry out what they have agreed to do. Don't be surprised or discouraged if an individual says they have not been able to put the performance they have agreed into practice. Why do you think this happens?

When you engage in mindful coaching, check out with each person how likely it is that they can and will put into practice what you have both agreed. If you don't, you will have created the illusion that 'all is well' and going ahead when, instead, you have created an additional problem. Therefore, you must consider the factors which may block or inhibit the person putting an agreed performance into practice.

You need to ask yourself some critical questions.

- Has this person got what it takes to produce the performance we have decided and agreed?

- Have they got the necessary commitment, skills and competence?

- Are we clear about what we mean by performance and the form it will take?

- What results do we expect to see, hear, observe, find or record that will clearly indicate that the agreed performance is being carried through into action?

These questions are all mindful coaching questions for the individual who wants to, and is motivated to, improve their concentration. More than this, they are signposts for both the coach and the individual – signposts that point to the need for a growing self-evaluation by the individual.

Awareness and responsibility

Here the concentration mindful coaching objective is to raise the individual's awareness and ability to take responsibility for their performance and behaviours. This is often gained by using effective active listening and questioning techniques. Telling generates resistance. Awareness and responsibility are raised by asking, guiding and facilitating the individual's learning, rather than by telling them what to do and how it should be done. The former can quickly lead to disengagement by the individual. The latter encourages the individual to develop awareness, personal responsibility and engagement in their own learning.

❖ **Awareness is knowing what is happening around you.**

❖ **Self-awareness is knowing what you are experiencing.**

❖ **Responsibility is where people own *their* choices.**

❖ **Personal responsibility is owning the choices we make.**

In attempting to increase an individual's awareness and to take personal responsibility, the coach might adopt the position of 'naive enquirer', rather than making pronouncements, because these can be perceived as threatening. For example, if you state, 'You're responsible for this ...', it can come across as a veiled threat, as opposed to a comment such as, 'How confident do you feel you can finish this on time? What, if any, obstacles do you see in the way of you achieving this?'

Clearly, facilitating the individual's learning, their self-awareness and personal responsibility can be enhanced by asking appropriate questions.

Asking appropriate questions

Asking questions is central to the mindful coaching of individuals with concentration difficulties. However, 'Why?' questions should be asked very seldom, if at all. A major reason for this is, 'Why?' questions can lead the individual to provide answers they may not know to be true, yet feel expected to give an answer, any answer. Pursuing 'Why?' questions with the individual also runs the risk of leading to a 'theory' about the individual, when what the individual needs is this information, which can be recapped, evaluated and on which they can take action.

Coaches need to obtain relevant information about the individual's concentration and clarify how difficulties in concentration can be improved. Clarifying concentration difficulties can be done well by the coach, and the individual, asking relevant, open questions such as 'What, when, who, which, where and how?'

As mindful coaching progresses, the individual can begin to see this approach as a model to adopt for themselves. The coach models the questions and evaluations which the individual can then progressively use, becoming their own coach. Where this works well, the individual can still work in collaboration with the coach, but engages more in self-questioning. This is a step towards developing self-mindful coaching.

Examples of mindful coaching questions

What questions

- What difficulties are you aware of?

- What solutions have you tried already?

- What works best for you?

- What gets in the way of listening to me or other people?

- What helps you to listen more to me or other people?

- What are you thinking when you have this problem?

- What are you thinking when you don't have this problem?

- What are you feeling when you don't have this problem?

- What are you doing that prevents you from focusing on the task?

- What are you doing that helps you to focus on the task?

When questions

- When are these difficulties present?

- When are these problems absent?

- When does this solution not work?

- When does this solution work?

- When do you not listen well?

- When do you listen best?

- When does your thinking get in the way of concentrating?

Speechmark

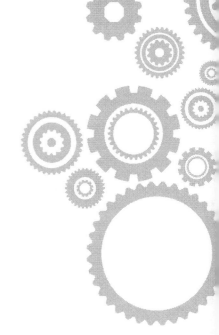

- When does your thinking focus your mind?

- When do your feelings create problems for you?

- When do your feelings help you to concentrate?

- When does what you are doing interfere with the task?

- What does what you are doing help you focus on the task?

Who questions

- Who is present when you have these difficulties?

- Who is present when this is not a problem?

- Who is present when this solution does not work for you?

- Who is present when this solution works for you?

- Who do you listen to best?

- Who do you not listen to?

- Who interrupts or stops your thinking?

- Who helps you to start or keep thinking?

- Who gives you feelings that create problems for you?

- Who gives you feelings that help you to concentrate?

- Who stops you doing what you need to do on the task?

- Who enables you to do what you are doing and helps you focus on the task?

Which questions

- Which tasks can you concentrate on the best?

- Which tasks make it difficult for you to concentrate?

- Which way makes it easier for you to listen?

- Which way makes it hard for you to listen?

- Which tasks interest you most?

- Which tasks interest you least?

Speechmark Ⓢ

- Which tasks help you to think?

- Which tasks

Where questions

- Where do you concentrate well?

- Where is it difficult for you to concentrate?

- Where is it easier for you to listen?

- Where is it hard for you to listen?

- Where do tasks interest you most?

- Where do tasks not interest you?

- Where is the best place for you to think?

- Where do you find thinking difficult?

- Where do you feel relaxed or alert?

- Where do you feel under stress or unable to relax?

- Where do you feel you concentrate the best?

- Where do your feelings get in the way of concentrating?

How questions

- How are these difficulties present?

- How are these problems absent?

- How does this solution not work?

- How does this solution work?

- How do you listen the least?

- How do you listen the best?

- How does your thinking get in the way of concentrating?

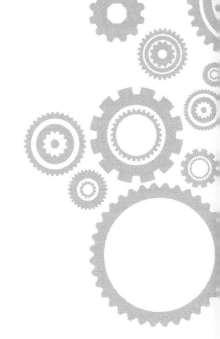

- How does your thinking help you focus your mind?

- How do your feelings create problems for you?

- How do your feelings help you to concentrate?

- How does what you are doing interfere with the task?

- How does what you are doing help you focus on the task?

Examples of self-mindful coaching questions

What questions

- What difficulties am I aware of?

- What solutions have I tried already?

- What works best for me?

- What gets in the way of me listening to myself or other people?

- What helps me to listen more to myself or other people?

- What am I thinking when I have this problem?

- What am I thinking when I don't have this problem?

- What am I feeling when I don't have the problem?

- What am I doing that prevents me from focusing on the task?

- What am I doing that helps me to focus on the task?

When questions

- When are these difficulties present for me?

- When are these problems absent for me?

- When does this solution not work for me?

- When does this solution work for me?

- When do I listen the least?

- When do I listen the best?

- When does my thinking get in the way of concentrating?

- When does my thinking help focus my mind?

- When do my feelings create problems for me?

- When do my feelings help me to concentrate?

- When does what I am doing interfere with the task?

- When does what I am doing help me focus on the task?

Who questions

- Who is present when I have these difficulties?

- Who is present when this is not a problem for me?

- Who is present when this solution does not work for me?

- Who is present when this solution works for me?

- Who do I listen to the best?

- Who don't I listen to?

- Who interrupts or stops me thinking?

- Who helps me to start or keep thinking?

- Who gives me feelings that create problems for me?

- Who gives me feelings that help me to concentrate?

- Who stops me doing what I need to do on the task?

- Who enables me to do what I am doing and helps me focus on the task?

Which questions

- Which tasks or activities can I concentrate on the best?

- Which tasks or activities make it difficult for me to concentrate?

- Which way makes it easier for me to listen?

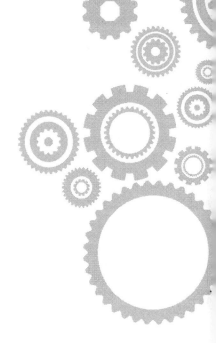

- Which way makes it hard for me to listen?

- Which tasks or activities interest me the most?

- Which tasks or activities interest me the least?

- Which tasks or activities help me to think?

- Which tasks or activities block my thinking?

- Which tasks or activities make me feel good?

- Which tasks or activities make me feel bad?

- Which feelings help me to concentrate?

- Which feelings stop me concentrating?

Where questions

- Where do I concentrate well?

- Where is it difficult for me to concentrate?

- Where is it easier for me to listen?

- Where do I find it hard to listen?

- Where do tasks interest me the most?

- Where do tasks not interest me?

- Where is the best place for me to think?

- Where do I find thinking difficult?

- Where do I feel relaxed or alert?

- Where do I feel under stress or unable to relax?

- Where do I feel I concentrate best?

- Where do my feelings get in the way of concentrating?

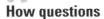

How questions

- How are these difficulties present for me?

- How are these problems absent for me?

- How does this solution not work for me?

- How does this solution work for me?

- How do I manage to not listen?

- How do I manage to listen the best?

- How does my thinking get in the way of my concentrating?

- How does my thinking help me to focus my mind?

- How do my feelings create problems for me?

- How do my feelings help me to concentrate better?

- How does what I am doing interfere with the task?

- How does what I am doing help me to focus on the task?

Advancing understanding

Through establishing rapport and trust, facilitative learning, increasing awareness and asking appropriate questions, the coach can lead the individual towards fresh insights, self-evaluation and learning. These work together in empowering the individual towards advancing their understanding of their concentration difficulties and how they might be improved.

A fundamental task the individual has to face is to overcome any emotional insecurity or other psychological blocks which prevent them from improving their concentration. However, the individual should not have to face this task entirely on their own. It is a task *the coach and the individual* need to face together. In this way, the individual feels supported and understood.

To advance understanding, the coach can help the individual in the following ways.

- *Identifying and making connections* between the way they receive information and how this contributes to, or interferes with, their concentration.

- *Identifying any themes or patterns of their thinking* that either augment or impair concentration in some way.

  Speechmark

- *Maintaining helpful behaviours* which may be useful to the individual or the people who obstruct them in improving their concentration.

- *Changing unhelpful behaviours* which may be problematic to the individual or the people who obstruct them in improving their concentration.

- *Sharing hunches and alternative interpretations* about the individual's concentration difficulties with them and how they could learn to concentrate better.

- *Challenging inconsistencies in the individual's knowledge and evaluation* of their concentration difficulties and how they could be better managed or improved.

- *Confronting unhelpful beliefs* which the individual may hold that cause or maintain blocks to the progress they can make in better understanding their concentration and how it can be improved.

- *Self-disclosing their feelings and experiences* which might help the individual learn from or identify similar feelings and experiences they are having.

- *Sharing information with the individual* to facilitate a climate in which the individual learns to increase their knowledge and reduce their ignorance about their concentration difficulties and misplaced assumptions about concentration: eg 'I will never be able to concentrate', 'I can't concentrate'.

Evaluating, reflecting and planning further action

The overall aim of mindful coaching is to help the individual to develop critical self-evaluation and self-reflection skills. Initially, however, the coach shows the individual how this can be done. In this model of mindful coaching, the individual learns to evaluate and reflect on how they receive information, and their thinking, feelings and behaviours as these pertain to concentration. To do this, the coach models to the individual the core skills of evaluating, reflecting and planning for future action. The individual can then adopt and adapt these, so they can continue to understand and improve their concentration without always depending on the coach.

In mindful coaching of the individual, the coach is seen as a linking 'bridge'. Here the individual learns, through the coach, to 'cross the bridge' and start:

- reflecting on the progress made

- identifying areas that still need work

- exploring strategies for maintaining the progress already made, and identifying any people who may be of help

- setting realistic goals or outcomes required

- evaluating any possible blocks to progress and exploring ways of overcoming them

- celebrating success

- planning for the future.

Developing concentration skills

Mindful coaching also includes empowering the individual to acquire, build and learn concentration skills. Here the emphasis is often on facilitating improvements in performance on a task. For this to happen, the individual may also need to develop new concentration skills as well as maintaining and improving their existing ones.

Improving concentration and subsequent performance on a task is not just a matter of thinking. It also requires dedicated rehearsal, a commitment to training the mind, and the regular practice of concentration skills. At these points in mindful coaching, the coach should inspire and encourage the individual by helping them to imagine how they will think and feel learning new concentration skills that lead to improved performance.

During this process, some individuals may become unsure of themselves and experience feelings of doubt in their ability to learn new concentration skills or improve their concentration. However, where this happens, the coach should convey to the individual that feeling doubt and uncertainty is often a normal reaction to change. The overriding attitude of the coach should be one of believing in the individual, demonstrating encouragement, and communicating that they can learn to strengthen their existing concentration skills and learn new ones.

By conveying an unwavering belief in the individual, the coach can increase the individual's self-confidence and inspire their efforts at improving their existing skills and in learning new concentration skills.

(Bailey & Brown, 2012)

Enhancing existing concentration skills and acquiring new ones may be developed through different pathways and procedures. Working with our approach to mindful coaching, the coach aims to facilitate individual learning by explaining methods and models and sharing ideas with them which have been shown to help other people. In our model, the coach is also encouraged to give useful feedback and to model to the individual appropriate, constructive and positive ways of evaluating their concentration and how it could be improved.

At times, this means the coach works with the individual to become SMART: helping them to set **S**pecific, **M**easurable, **A**chievable, **R**ealistic and **T**ime-bound goals. At other times, the coach will be less specific, emphasising active rehearsal, distraction management, and the development of increased self-evaluation, and competency in concentration. In our experience, combining mindful coaching with training in relevant concentration skills increases the likelihood of each individual improving their concentration.

PART 3

Concentration skills training

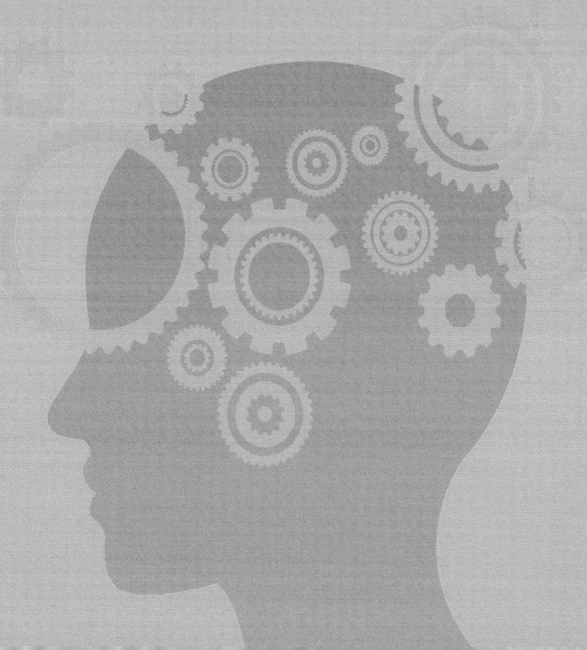

Introduction

The activities in this part of the resource book are specially designed to help you understand and improve your concentration skills.

Each activity has been used and developed further by the authors. They reflect the wide range of activities that are considered helpful in enhancing concentration skills.

We have coded the activities in the Concentration Activity Guide (CAG) below. This shows you which aspect of concentration the activity aims to improve. Some of the CAG activities target all five domains of concentration. Others are more specific in their design and focus on just one or two target domains.

Concentration Activity Guide

Activity no and title	Domain of concentration				
	Receiving	Thinking	Feeling/emotions	Doing	Environment
1 Being aware	✓	✓	✓	✓	✓
2 Mindful breathing	✓	✓	✓	✓	✓
3 Concentration bubbles	✓	✓	✓	✓	✓
4 Cultivating patience		✓	✓		
5 Just sitting, just breathing	✓	✓	✓	✓	✓
6 Walking concentration	✓	✓	✓	✓	✓
7 Mind freeing		✓			
8 Racquet and ball	✓			✓	✓
9 Keys to concentration	✓	✓	✓	✓	✓
10 Silence in concentration	✓	✓	✓	✓	✓
11 Tracking concentration	✓	✓	✓	✓	✓
12 Visual focusing	✓	✓	✓	✓	✓
13 Concentration span	✓			✓	
14 Facilitators and distractors	✓	✓	✓	✓	✓
15 Building resistance to distraction				✓	✓

Activity no and title	Domain of concentration				
	Receiving	Thinking	Feeling/emotions	Doing	Environment
16 Guiding concentration through self-talk		✓	✓		
17 Getting unstuck through visualisation		✓	✓		
18 Emotional stress distractors			✓	✓	
19 Doing concentration		✓			✓
20 Being in the flow	✓	✓	✓	✓	✓
21 Modes of concentration	✓	✓	✓	✓	✓
22 Achieving optimal alertness states		✓		✓	✓
23 Alertness states			✓	✓	✓
24 Getting started on a task: overcoming resistance		✓			✓
25 Getting started on a task: 'warming up'		✓			✓
26 Switching attention	✓	✓			
27 Concentration force field		✓	✓		
28 Active listening	✓	✓	✓	✓	
29 Listening tree	✓				
30 Motivation: raising awareness	✓	✓			
31 Motivation: when interest level is low	✓	✓			✓
32 Motivation: not in the mood			✓		
33 Motivation: rewards				✓	
34 Motivation: environment				✓	✓
35 Motivation: conflicting motives		✓			✓

Activity 1 | Being aware

Introduction

Taming the wandering mind begins with being aware. Our awareness is moving and dynamic. Most of the time, we are not aware of our body postures, movements, actions, thoughts, feelings and behaviours. Usually this is not a bad thing because we have come to rely on our learned behaviour, which usually works well for us. For example, leaning over and lifting a chair is something we do not have to think about. It has become a useful behaviour that we engage in occasionally whenever a chair has to be lifted.

Many of our learned behaviours have become habits that we rely on in our daily lives. However, starting to improve our concentration is assisted when we intentionally become aware of our body, mind, feelings and behaviour.

Purpose

To centre your mind and become more aware of your body, mind, feelings and behaviour.

Resources

• Personal journal

What to do

1 Sit in an armchair.

2 Keep your back straight.

3 Your arms should be supported by the armchair or on your lap.

4 Close your eyes.

Now begin your progressive awareness activity by working through the following steps.

5 I am aware of my feet.

6 I am aware of my legs.

7 I am aware of my arms.

8 I feel my breathing in.

9 I feel my breathing out.

10 I experience my body in the chair.

11 I feel my body touching the chair.

12 I am aware of my listening.

13 I am aware of listening to my listening.

14 I feel my stillness.

15 I experience calming in my mind.

16 I am aware of feeling relaxed.

17 I am aware of my thinking.

18 I am aware of thinking about my thinking.

19 I am aware of being calm and focused.

20 I am aware of being aware.

21 Make notes in your personal journal about what you are learning about being aware of concentration and your thoughts, feelings and behaviour.

22 Regularly practise and review being aware and note how changes in your habits can help to tame a wandering mind.

Coaching evaluation

Evaluate being aware and your learning with your coach. When you have increased being aware and become able to self-evaluate, you can also do this yourself and become your own inner coach.

Once you can do this, you can practise being aware in other situations, for example:

- Having a conversation

- Reading a book

- Going for a walk

- Listening to music

- Looking at an object

- Gazing at the stars

- Listening to birdsong or the sound of waves

  Speechmark

- Watching the movement of your body

- Listening to what another person is saying

- Choosing what you say and how you say it.

Notes

Activity 2 | Mindful breathing

Introduction

We are breathing all of the time. Yet we are usually unaware of it. We could not live our lives if we were continuously aware of our breathing. However, by adopting a mindful approach to our breathing, we can select times to practise it and improve our concentration.

Being mindful of our breathing is simply being aware of it and not getting in the way of it. This means letting any distracting thoughts, feelings or movements happen and watching them coming and going as they arise in our mind and then allowing them to depart. All we have to do is be aware and keep our mind focused on our breathing.

Purpose

To increase your ability to direct attention.

Resources

- Chair

- Paper or a flipchart

What to do

1   Stop what you are doing.

2   Sit down and focus all your attention on your nose.

3   Do this by keeping your eyes open and focusing on the end of your nose.

4   Pay attention to the air going in and out of your nose.

5   Just notice – let it happen all by itself (don't try to force it or make it happen).

6   Let any thoughts that arise come and go, like waves disappearing on the seashore.

7   After a few moments, close your eyes and now feel the air going in and out through your nose.

8   Keep following your breathing for a few minutes.

9   Let all thoughts, images, sounds and feelings come and go.

10 Now open your eyes, turn your attention to your surroundings and notice what you see and hear.

11 Keep doing this for a few more moments.

12 End your session by taking three deep breaths and return to what you were doing.

Coaching evaluation

Evaluate your experience and learning intentions with your coach ,or self-evaluate.

Issues to consider in your coaching evaluation

*   What did you notice most about your mindful breathing?

*   How did it feel?

*   What thoughts helped or hindered your session?

*   What was the best part of this session for you?

*   What was the worst part?

*   How could you benefit from doing more mindful breathing?

Notes

_____

_____

_____

_____

_____

_____

_____

_____

_____

_____

_____

_____

_____

_____

_____

_____

_____

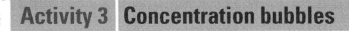

Activity 3 | Concentration bubbles

Introduction

Some people can develop a deep state of concentration. They often describe this state as being in a 'concentration bubble'. Many high achievers in education, business and sport and in their interpersonal relationships can create this concentration bubble. They do this for different tasks they have to carry out. Some people can create a concentration bubble and stay in it for short periods of time. Others manage, with practice, to stay in their concentration bubble for longer periods of time.

Purpose

This activity shows you how to create your own concentration bubble and practise staying in it.

Resources

• Concentration bubbles graphic (page 64)

What to do

1 Start by imagining a time when you can concentrate really well.

2 Note what helps you to do this most. For example, is it sitting still or is it moving, such as walking, or listening to music, or looking at and focusing on a visual image?

3 Find out what works best for you.

4 When you have done this, write it down or make a drawing of it inside the concentration bubbles on page 64.

5 End your session by reflecting on and rehearsing in your mind what helps you extend your concentration.

Coaching evaluation

Evaluate your experience and learning intentions with your coach, or self-evaluate.

Issues to consider in your coaching evaluation

• What did you notice when you were doing this activity?

• How long did you manage to stay in this state of concentration?

• When do you think you might use this approach?

Notes

_____

_____

_____

_____

_____

_____

_____

_____

_____

_____

_____

_____

_____

_____

_____

_____

_____

_____

_____

_____

_____

Speechmark

Concentration Bubbles

Speechmark

Activity 4 | Cultivating patience

Introduction

Having patience with ourselves and other people is not always easy. Also, being patient when we are concentrating on a task contributes to our being able to stay on task and complete what we are trying to do.

Learning to develop patience also helps us counter impatience. When we can do this, it prevents our own impatience, undermining our concentration.

Being more patient assists us in receiving information, thinking more clearly and not becoming frustrated so much that it 'hijacks' what we are concentrating on.

Purpose

To understand how frustration affects your level of patience.

Resources

- Cultivating patience inventory (see page 67)

What to do

Becoming frustrated and losing your patience prevents you from concentrating. When you are concentrating, if you become frustrated and impatient, it can interrupt your concentration and your concentration 'breaks down'. Cultivating patience makes it less likely that your concentration will break down and increases you likelihood you can improve and maintain your concentration.

1 Recall a situation where you were very patient. Now start to notice what it was about yourself that allowed you to be patient.

2 Begin by looking at the postures and movements of your body and hands.

3 Study the postures and movements closely and copy them until you feel they are the same.

4 Next look at the breathing you did when you were patient and start breathing in that way now.

5 Say to yourself 'I am clear, calm and concentrating' and keep this going, bringing your posture, movements, rhythmical breathing and self-statements together.

6 When you have brought all of these features together, and they feel natural, complete the cultivating patience inventory on page 67. Use this as your reference point for how well

Speechmark

you are managing to be patient in situations that may be frustrating and interfere with your concentration.

7 End the session by making a commitment to keep your inventory up to date.

8 Continue practising cultivating patience for those situations you have to face in the future that may make demands on your patience.

Coaching evaluation

Evaluate your experience and learning intentions with your coach, or self-evaluate.

Issues to consider in your coaching evaluation

• What did you learn about your patience, frustration and concentration?

• How did your feelings alter?

• In which situations are you more, or less, patient?

• In what way do you think this knowledge and experience might be useful for you?

Notes

CULTIVATING PATIENCE INVENTORY

Complete the Cultivating Patience Inventory (CPI) below, noting those situations where you are patient and impatient, how your body behaves, the postures you adopt and the way you speak to yourself and feel in these situations. When you have done this, reflect on what you have learned and make a personal commitment to how you will cultivate and strengthen your patience.

Situations where I am patient	Situations where I am impatient	My body movement	My posture	Breathing	How I speak to myself	How I feel

My commitment to cultivating patience

_____

_____

_____

_____

_____

Name: _____ **Date:** _____

Activity 5 Just sitting, just breathing

Introduction

Sometimes we are so busy rushing around that we are unable to concentrate. We are so busy, we forget to slow down and simply be calm and let our concentration return.

To improve our concentration, all we have to do is to learn to sit still and focus on our posture and breathing. When we just sit and just breathe, we learn to train our wandering mind.

Purpose

To develop calmness and focused attention.

Resources

• Personal learning journal

What to do

1 Sit in a comfortable chair.

2 Adopt an upright posture.

3 Don't lean back or forward.

4 Keep your back straight.

5 Now take a few deep breaths.

6 Say 'calm' to yourself as you breathe out.

7 Become aware of your body in the chair.

8 Notice your breathing.

9 Notice each inward breath.

10 And with each outward breath, experience the sense of letting go.

11 Let any stray thoughts come and go.

12 Become even more aware of your breathing.

13 Notice you are aware of just sitting, just breathing.

14 Let your concentration return and be fully aware of each moment.

15 Just be present – mindful of just sitting – just breathing.

16 Let it all happen – nothing to do – just fully concentrate.

17 End the session by taking a few deep breaths and returning to what you were doing.

Coaching evaluation

Evaluate your experience and learning intentions with your coach, or self-evaluate.

Issues to consider in your coaching evaluation

- What did you notice when you were just sitting, just breathing?

- How far were these things arising from inside your mind or outside it?

- Which events had the most effect?

- How much did they come and go?

- What benefits or drawbacks does just sitting and just breathing have for you?

Notes

_____

_____

_____

_____

_____

_____

_____

_____

_____

_____

_____

_____

_____

_____

_____

_____

_____

_____

_____

_____

Activity 6 | Walking concentration
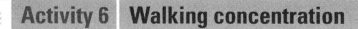

Introduction

Walking is something we take for granted. We do not go through each day paying any attention to our walking. Yet when we do become focused on our walking, we can increase our mental muscle – our ability to improve our concentration.

Practising walking concentration is a simple but powerful way to increase the quality of our concentration as well as the amount of time we can stay focused on particular tasks.

Purpose

To improve the quality of your concentration.

Resources

• Walking shoes

What to do

1 Decide to go for a walk for 10–15 minutes.

2 Sit on a chair and put on a pair of walking shoes.

3 Right away, be aware of the movements you make putting on your shoes.

4 Focus your awareness on standing up and walking out of the door.

5 At this point, simply be conscious of the movements of your legs.

6 Now maintain your focus and be aware of each step you take.

7 Follow this by alternating your attention between each step you take.

8 Continue by focusing on the left, right, left, right, left, right rhythmic motion of your legs and feet.

9 Stay in the awareness of every single moment and the movement of the steps you take.

10 Notice only the movement in each moment.

11 Carry on like this throughout your walking, being aware only of each movement you make.

12 Begin finishing your walking concentration by returning to the chair once more.

13 Focus on slowly removing your walking shoes.

14 End by taking three deep breaths through your nose and breathing out through your mouth.

15 Now go and spend some time on a task requiring your full concentration.

Coaching evaluation

Evaluate your experience and learning intentions with your coach, or self-evaluate.

Issues to consider in your coaching evaluation

- Reflect on your walking concentration.

- Explore and evaluate where and when it worked best and least.

- What would help improve your focus during walking concentration?

- How might you do that?

Notes

_____

_____

_____

_____

_____

_____

_____

_____

_____

_____

_____

_____

_____

_____

_____

_____

_____

_____

_____

_____

Activity 7 | Mind freeing

Introduction

Sometimes we get caught up in rigid thinking. At these times, we believe we cannot concentrate. Believing this only reinforces our rigid thinking. Rigid thinking is habit of mind – a bad habit.

However, just as we can get into thinking habits that block or interfere with our concentration, so too we can develop flexible thinking. Flexible thinking frees our mind to generate new ways of thinking and improving our concentration.

Purpose

This activity aims to facilitate mind freeing so that you can develop more flexible thinking and make progress in concentrating.

Resources

• Pens and paper

What to do

1 Draw a square.

2 Look carefully at it and note the length and shape of the lines.

3 Now draw a circle inside the square. Again study the shape of the line.

4 Next place a dot inside the circle and be aware of the shape of it.

5 Look at the shapes you have created and close your eyes.

6 Imagine how the three shapes keep changing form, eg one might be bigger or smaller or different in colour from the others, or think of them as words you can see or hear.

7 Allow this to happen and go with the flow of these changes in your mind.

8 Open your eyes and immediately draw the images or write the words you saw or heard.

9 Don't hold back – just let any images and words come to mind.

10 Notice how you have freed your mind to think more flexibly and yet still concentrate.

11 Complete the activity again but this time only in your mind.

12 End by reflecting on how well you have done in freeing your thinking and improving your concentration.

Coaching evaluation

Evaluate your experience and learning intentions with your coach, or self-evaluate.

Issues to consider in your coaching evaluation

- Assess those tasks where your thinking can block your performance.

- Explore how mind freeing might help you to free your thinking about a specific task.

- Monitor your concentration over the next week and note down any time when your thinking becomes blocked for any reason.

- Consider using this mind-freeing exercise at these and other times when your mind needs to be free from distraction.

Notes

_____

_____

_____

_____

_____

_____

_____

_____

_____

_____

_____

_____

_____

_____

_____

_____

_____

Activity 8 | Racquet and ball (building your concentration muscle)

Introduction

One of the appealing things about concentration is that we can learn to increase our 'mental strength'. Increasing the length of time we can concentrate is like building our 'concentration muscle'. When we can do this, we can also sustain our concentration on tasks over longer periods of time.

We can learn to increase the amount of time we concentrate by carrying out activities that require us to combine movement with focused visual attention. As well as helping you to build your 'concentration muscle', this activity is fun to do.

Purpose

To improve your ability to concentrate while you are moving.

Resources

- Tennis racquet
- Tennis ball
- Stopwatch (optional)

What to do

1   Find a space where you are free to move around.

2   Pick up the tennis racquet and ball.

3   Hold the racquet in your preferred hand.

4   Place the tennis ball on top of the racquet.

5   Now do a trial to get used to the task and start bouncing the tennis ball upwards on top of the racquet.

6   Focus on what you are doing, make any movements with your wrist or body that help you to keep the ball bouncing up and down on top of the racquet.

7   When you have done this, repeat the task, this time counting how many times you can keep the ball bouncing up and down on the racquet.

8   When the ball falls off the racquet, write down the number you managed to reach, eg 5, 10, 15, 20, 25.

9   Repeat the task and see whether you can increase the number of times you keep the ball bouncing.

10 A variation of this task is to start a stopwatch before each time you do the task and stop it when the ball falls off the racquet.

Speechmark

11 This gives you an idea of how long you can stay focused on the task as well as how many times you can keep the tennis ball bouncing on the racquet.

12 End the session by reviewing your record of how long you kept focused on the task and the number of times you kept the ball bouncing up and down on the racquet.

Coaching evaluation

Evaluate your experience and learning intentions with your coach, or self-evaluate.

Issues to consider in your coaching evaluation

- How easy was it for you to focus visually?
- How difficult was it for you to focus visually?
- How easy was it for you to concentrate on movement?
- How difficult was it for you to concentrate on movement?
- How easy was it for you to concentrate on combining visual concentration and movement?
- How difficult was it for you to concentrate on combining visual concentration and movement?
- What can you do to build your 'concentration muscle'?

Notes

_____

_____

_____

_____

_____

_____

_____

_____

_____

_____

_____

_____

_____

Activity 9 | Keys to concentration

Introduction

When we are concentrating well, everything seems to be in the 'right place'. We receive information, listen and attend in a focused way. We think clearly and keep our mind on the task at hand. We do things that are in keeping with the demands of the task. We are able to keep unwanted and intrusive emotional stress from disrupting our concentration.

Being in the 'right place' with concentration is as if a key has unlocked our ability to concentrate. Identifying, mapping and rehearsing our keys to concentration is a useful activity because these 'keys' help us to unlock and improve our concentration.

Purpose

To learn how to trigger good concentration.

Resources

- Keys to concentration map (page 78)

- Pens and paper

What to do

1   Recall a time when you were able to concentrate.

2   Notice your surroundings and what you were focusing on.

3   Now bring back what you were thinking at the time.

4   Now run those thoughts through your mind again and really 'capture' those thoughts.

5   Recall how you were feeling and let those feelings come back to you right now.

6   When you've got those feelings again, join the thoughts you had along with those feelings.

7   Replay these together now – the thoughts with the feelings, and the feelings with the thoughts.

8   Do this five to ten times in your mind.

9   Write down, or draw on your keys to concentration map (page 78), what you were focusing on, receiving, thinking, feeling and doing and the surroundings you were in.

10 End by rehearsing your focusing, thinking, feelings, doing, your 'best' surroundings, and how you can use these keys to concentrate on future tasks.

Coaching evaluation

Evaluate your experience and learning intentions with your coach, or self-evaluate.

Issues to consider in your coaching evaluation

- What is your receiving information key to improving your concentration?

- What is your thinking key to improving your concentration?

- What is your doing key to improving your concentration?

- What is your emotional key to improving your concentration?

- What is your environment key to improving your concentration?

- How can you link all these keys to unlock the power of your concentration?

Notes

_____

_____

_____

_____

_____

_____

_____

_____

_____

_____

_____

_____

_____

_____

_____

_____

_____

_____

Speechmark

Keys to concentration map

Write down or draw your keys to concentration below. Show what you were focusing on, receiving, thinking, feeling and doing and the surroundings you were in at the time.

--- **Focusing on**

--- **Receiving**

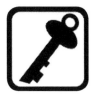

--- **Thinking**

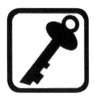

--- **Feeling**

--- **Doing**

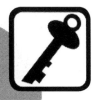

--- **Environment**

Activity 10 | Silence in concentration

Introduction

We can improve our concentration by increasing the amount of time we can be silent. Being able to sit in silence is in itself a disciplined form of concentration. When we are silent we can notice what is going on in our mind. We can see, hear, feel, think, be aware of all this and what we are doing and whether it helps or hinders our concentration. We can learn to let go of what hinders our concentration and bring into the present moment what helps it.

Developing silence in concentration takes practice. The more we practise silence in concentration, the better we can get at it, and lengthen the amount of time we can concentrate.

Purpose

To increase your capacity to concentrate over time.

Resources

- Stopwatch or the seconds hand on a watch or a clock, or an egg-timer

- Silence in concentration inventory and graph (page 81)

What to do

1   Set the stopwatch, or the seconds hand of the watch or clock, or the egg-timer for 10 seconds.

2   Close your eyes.

3   Now just focus on your breathing.

4   Notice your breath as it goes in and out of your body.

5   Feel it in moving in and out of your nostrils.

6   Try it out now and do a few practice breaths.

7   Stop immediately the clock alarm or timer rings.

8   Begin by adopting silence in concentration for a short time and build it up gradually (eg 10, 20, 30, 40, 50, 60 seconds).

9   Increase the amount of time you can do silence in concentration at 10-second intervals.

10 Only move on to increasing the amount of time you can spend in silent concentration when you have achieved a previous time (eg move from 20 to 30 seconds).

11 Do not try to skip a level (eg do not try to practise 50 seconds of silence in concentration if you have only been able to do 10 seconds).

12 End your session by completing the silence in concentration inventory and graph (see page 81).

Coaching evaluation

Evaluate your experience and learning intentions with your coach, or self-evaluate.

Issues to consider in your coaching evaluation

- What did you discover from trying silent concentration?

- What did you see, feel, hear and think?

- How far were you able to let go of what got in the way of silent concentration?

- How long did your awareness of silent concentration last?

- What are the best conditions for you to practise silent concentration?

Notes

_____

_____

_____

_____

_____

_____

_____

_____

_____

_____

_____

_____

_____

_____

_____

_____

_____

_____

 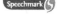

Silence in concentration inventory and graph

Keeping a record of silence in concentration allows you to see how far you can increase the length of time you can concentrate. Record your sessions and notice any patterns, eg whether you can sit in silence better in the morning, afternoon or evening.

Time (seconds)

120										
100										
90										
80										
70										
60										
50										
40										
30										
20										
10										
0										
Morning	1	2	3	4	5	6	7	8	9	10
Afternoon	1	2	3	4	5	6	7	8	9	10
Evening	1	2	3	4	5	6	7	8	9	10
Date/time of session										

Number of sessions

Name _____ Age _____

Activity 11 — Tracking concentration

Introduction

Concentration is something we take for granted so much that we often don't know what distracts us from concentrating or facilitates improvement in our concentration. How well we concentrate depends on five main domains relating to concentration:

1 the way we receive and attend to information

2 our thinking

3 our emotional status

4 what we are doing

5 the environment we are in at the time.

Distractors activated in any of these domains, or in different combinations, can disrupt and sometimes substantially impair our concentration. Mapping out the domains of concentration helps us to track when our concentration is being impaired and how we can improve it.

Purpose

To become aware of distractions to your concentration.

Resources

• Pens and a journal, notebook, or tablet/laptop

What to do

1 Say why concentration depends on limiting distractions and increasing the facilitation of domains of concentration.

Distractors

2 Recall a time or task(s) where you could not concentrate.

3 Break it down into the five domains of concentration.

4 How were you attending to and receiving information?

5 What were you thinking when you were not concentrating?

6 How were you feeling at the time (eg high, scared, angry)?

7 What were you doing at the time?

8 Map out the environment or surroundings you were in.

9 Record this in your journal, notebook, tablet or laptop.

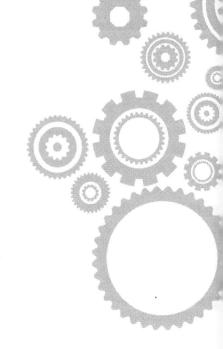

Facilitators

10 Identify a time when you could concentrate.

11 Again, break it down into the five domains of concentration.

12 How were you attending to and receiving information?

13 What were you thinking when you were concentrating?

14 How were you feeling at the time (eg relaxed, balanced, composed)?

15 What were you doing at the time?

16 Specify the environment or surroundings you were in.

17 End the session by recording what you have learned about tracking.

Coaching evaluation

Evaluate your experience and learning intentions with your coach, or self-evaluate.

Issues to consider in your coaching evaluation

• Which domains of concentration were you able to identify that improved or reduced your focus?

• How do you receive information that helps or hinders your concentration?

• What specifically do you do that helps or hinders your concentration?

• What are you thinking that helps or hinders your concentration?

• Which emotion(s) help you to improve or interfere with your concentration?

• Specifically, which settings facilitate or distract your concentration?

Notes

_____

_____

_____

_____

_____

_____

_____

_____

Activity 12 | Visual focusing

Introduction

Anyone who is trying to improve their concentration and performance can do so by acquiring the skill of visual focusing. Visual focusing means exactly what it says. We use our natural ability to visualise what we are doing in a way that it is clear and we focus all of our attention on that task or part of the task.

Visual focusing is a skill that we build up until it becomes second nature to us. Visual focusing is like learning to ride a bicycle. Once we have learned what to do, we only have to keep practising the skill to ensure we never forget it. Putting in place the building blocks that lead to greater visual focusing helps us in establishing and sustaining our concentration for longer periods of time.

Purpose

To develop and improve your visual concentration skills.

Resources

- Spiral graphic (see page 87)

- Circle graphic (see page 88)

What to do

Stage 1

1 Sit upright in a chair.

2 Adopt a comfortable position.

3 Rest your arms on your lap or on the arms of the chair.

4 Now become aware of the air going in and out of your nose.

5 With your eyes open, gaze at the image of the spiral for 1–5 minutes (on page 87).

6 Then close your eyes and see how long you can hold the image of the spiral before it fades.

7 Repeat the cycle of gazing at the spiral and closing your eyes. Do this a few times.

8 See if you were able to extend the amount of time you gazed at the spiral and held it in your mind.

Stage 2

9   Now, without gazing at the spiral, close your eyes and create a spiral image in your mind.

10 Begin focusing on the overall shape of the spiral and make it a size that suits you.

11 Continue being aware of the spiral and nothing else.

12 If you need to, you can sharpen up the image by opening your eyes and briefly gazing at the image of the spiral (on page 87) and closing your eyes again.

13 Keep doing this in your own time and at your own rate until you can create your inner image of a spiral.

14 As you become better at doing this, create your inner spiral and focus on rotating it in your mind, first clockwise then counterclockwise.

Stage 3

15 Repeat the visual focusing cycle. This time, gaze at the circle graphic (on page 88), close your eyes, and see how long you can maintain the image in your mind.

16 When you can do this, keep your eyes closed and imagine the black circle changing into a white circle on black paper and back again to a black circle on white paper. Notice what happens.

17 End your visual focusing session by taking a deep breath, stretching and opening your eyes.

Coaching evaluation

Evaluate your experience and learning intentions with your coach, or self-evaluate.

Issues to consider in your coaching evaluation

- What was the easiest or most difficult part of visual focusing for you?
- Which environment helps you to get the best out of visual focusing?
- How long were you able to concentrate and hold the spiral image in your mind?
- When you focused on moving the spiral image, what happened?
- How long were you able to visualise and focus on the black circle on the white paper?
- Were there any changes when you reversed this and made it a white circle on black paper?
- What happened to your concentration during visual focusing?
- How best can you use visual focusing to improve your concentration?

Notes

Speechmark Ⓢ

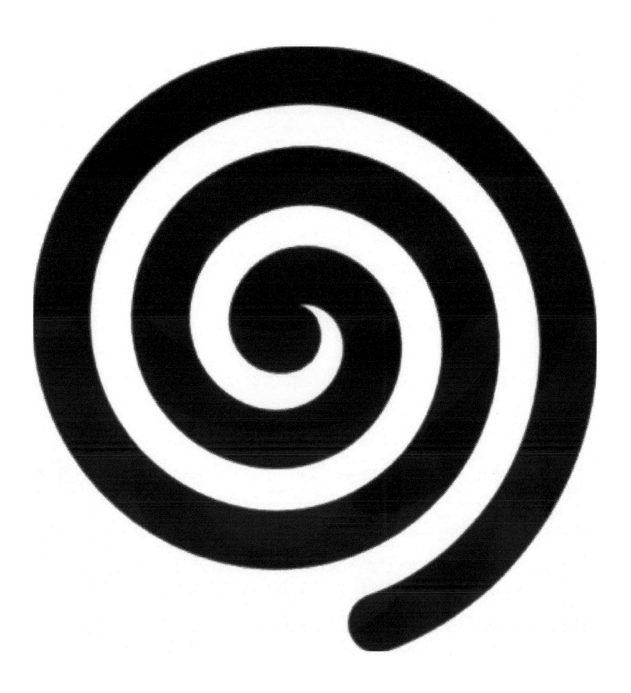

87

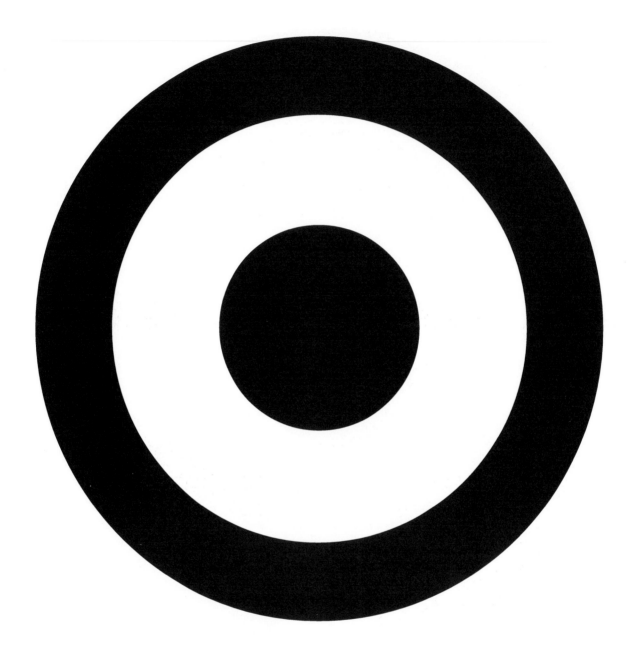

Clock face record

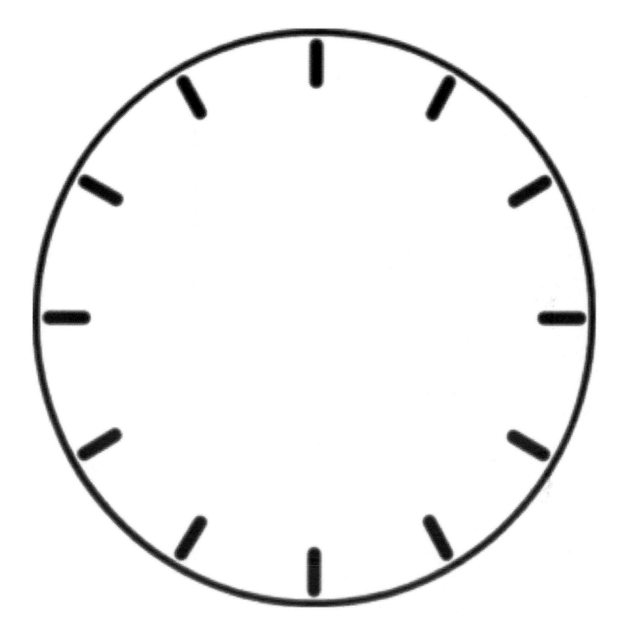

Activity 14　Facilitators and distractors

Introduction

Psychologists have shown how facilitators and distractors are important in influencing concentration and human performance. Facilitators are those situations or environmental conditions that really do contribute to your concentration. Distractors are those situations and environmental conditions that interfere with and undermine your concentration, either preventing you from concentrating or interrupting your concentration.

There are many kinds of facilitators and distractors. They can range from your state of mind and emotions at the time to different sounds and sights in your surroundings. Each person has their own facilitators and distractors. For example, one person may like playing music and this helps them to concentrate. Another may find music acts as a distractor, preventing them from concentrating or interrupting their concentration.

Clearly, one person's facilitator is another's distractor. Therefore, it is helpful to map your profile of individual facilitators and distractors. It can be useful in helping you to create the conditions whereby you can increase the presence of your facilitators and, at the same time, reduce or remove distractors that you find adversely affect your concentration.

Purpose

To identify personal facilitators and distractors and to develop the skills for managing them.

What to do

1　Describe and write down any facilitators that help you in concentrating.

2　Keep a record of how your facilitators actually help you to concentrate, maintain your concentration, or allow you to switch from one thing to another and keep your concentration.

3　Now describe and write down any distractors that interfere with or prevent you from concentrating.

4　Also keep a record of how your distractors adversely affect your concentration, such as breaking it up, preventing you from concentrating or stopping you from switching your concentration from one thing to another.

5　Now map your facilitators and distractors of concentration onto a whiteboard or flipchart, or in a personal 'concentration journal'.

6　One useful way of capturing this concentration personal data is to draw a line down the centre of the page, creating two columns, one headed 'Facilitators' and the other 'Distractors'.

7　Keep this journal up to date and discuss it with your coach.

8   You can also learn and apply self-evaluation and discover what you are doing or will do that increases the effects of facilitators of concentration in your life and decreases the influence of distractors.

9   Finally, make a facilitators and distractors concentration plan.

10 Decide how long you will practise your plan. Now put it into practice and decide when you will further evaluate with your coach, or self-evaluate, the facilitators and distractors affecting your concentration.

Coaching evaluation

Evaluate your experience and learning intentions with your coach, or self-evaluate.

Issues to consider in your coaching evaluation

- Which domains of concentration were you able to identify that improved or reduced your focus?

- How do you receive information that helps or hinders your concentration?

- What specifically do you do that helps or hinders your concentration?

- What are you thinking that helps or hinders your concentration?

- Which emotion(s) help you to improve or interfere with your concentration?

- Specifically, which settings facilitate or distract your concentration?

Notes

_____

_____

_____

_____

_____

_____

_____

_____

_____

_____

_____

_____

Activity 15 | Building resistance to distraction

Introduction

Most people can concentrate on tasks that are interesting, fun and motivating. It can be easy to concentrate on a task that is stimulating even if the task itself is quite challenging. A dull, repetitive activity may be less demanding but the mind can then become prone to distraction and wandering.

The hardest tasks for us to maintain a good focus on are often those which require minimal thought but quite high levels of attention. These may be tasks that do not interest us but ones that we cannot totally switch off from.

It can be useful to practise this type of task to build our ability to maintain a focus even when the task is comparatively straightforward.

Sustaining attention on a visually demanding yet repetitive task can build an individual's attention to detail.

Maintaining performance while being distracted can help to build an individual's resistance to distraction.

Purpose

This activity aims to help you to build resistance to distraction and your ability to work under pressure while performing a relatively undemanding visual-processing task.

Resources

- Numbers sheet (page 96)

- Letters sheet (page 97)

- For distraction – radio with talking, music or television programme

What to do

1 You will need as many activity sheets as required for the practice session.

2 Identify a target Number or Letter. Work through each sheet crossing out the Number or Letter you have selected.

3 Begin timing at the start of the task and stop timing when you have finished the sheet.

4 Repeat the exercise, trying to beat your time on the second run-through.

5 Introduce a distraction, eg radio, music, television programme.

6 Now repeat the timed exercise. This time, try to maintain your accuracy and speed by trying to ignore the distraction.

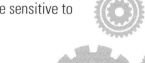

7   Try the exercise using different types of distraction and see whether you are more sensitive to any particular distraction.

8   Repeat as often as required to build resistance to distraction.

Coaching evaluation

Evaluate your experience and learning intentions with your coach, or self-evaluate.

Issues to consider in your coaching evaluation

- Did the timing of the activity affect your performance?

- How did you feel as the distractions were introduced and what impact did they have on your performance?

- Do you think you are more susceptible to verbal, musical or visual distractions?

- Consider what kind of distractions impact on your performance generally and think about how you can build your resistance.

Notes

_____

_____

_____

_____

_____

_____

_____

_____

_____

_____

_____

_____

14783927498375869504869582039282093475843923472837584928347918127472717282748379
28112892891839287483746576650129309029495787848928711232029302012102021012819894
38792857938479123163710290022540384039487982934592647126812152361576381749387487 8
78192831234524515632637264374270237120419293742093530945834004690340582837786481
72812532617823197298349875027598378783647167236715625137267698817287837182912879
28374029353453095409640564579305993845987987108237648273648273641238273489081792
38748741726482736427817236478135014957367826817139802752365384659128372494139579
18456328361862768176376134873487812768579014501854510211287381782718781817838178
1712321234231242342502199345235322354593849692113220192928198218918 9̀ 8̀ 9818812882
38271888181710047261587657236109824701147839274983758695048695820392820934758439
23472837584928347918127472717282748379281128928918392874837465766501293090294957
87848928711232029302012102021012819894387928579384791231637102902254038403948798
29345926471268121523615763817493874878781928312345245156326372643742702371204192
93742093530945834004690340582837786481728125326178231972983498750275983787836471
67236715625137267698817287837182912879283740293534530954096405645793059938459879
87108237648273648273641238273489081792387487417264827364278172364781350149573678
26817139802752365384659128372494139579184563283618627681763761348734878127685790
14501854510211287381782718781817838178171232123423124234250219934523532235459384
969211322019292819821891899̀ 8̀ 9818812882382718881817100472615876572361098247 01

fhoppojkdserttdfghyuj kuuu kmbfdpfre tgdcv ghjudfgry setrbcxdste
w bnmexfs d dafertyghjuukkrdsdf trr ylo oljy 5e ssdftt4 rll tr sfgh rfb
nkllppougdsd eewwrrtgfgfvbgtreddxcsfrfggthyfhbnjuytfrfvgaFhopp
ojkdserttdfghyuj kuuu kmbfdpfre tgdcv ghjudfgry setrbcxdstew bnm
exfs d dafertyghjuukkrdsdf trr ylo oljy 5e ssdftt4 rll tr sfgh rfbnkllpp
ougdsd eewwrrtgfgfvbgtreddxcsfrfggthyfhbnjuytfrfvgaFhoppojkdse
rttdfghyuj kuuu kmbfdpfre tgdcv ghjudfgry setrbcxdstew bnmexfs d
dafertyghjuukkrdsdf trr ylo oljy 5e ssdftt4 rll tr sfgh rfbnkllppougds
d eewwrrtgfgfvbgtreddxcsfrfggthyfhbnjuytfrfvgaFhoppojkdserttdfg
hyuj kuuu kmbfdpfre tgdcv ghjudfgry setrbcxdstew bnmexfs d dafert
yghjuukkrdsdf trr ylo oljy 5e ssdftt4 rll tr sfgh rfbnkllppougdsd eeww
rrtgfgfvbgtreddxcsfrfggthyfhbnjuytfrfvgaFhoppojkdserttdfghyuj ku
uu kmbfdpfre tgdcv ghjudfgry setrbcxdstew bnmexfs d dafertyghjuu
kkrdsdf trr ylo oljy 5e ssdftt4 rll tr sfgh rfbnkllppougdsd eewwrrtgfgf
vbgtreddxcsfrfggthyfhbnjuytfrfvgaFhoppojkdserttdfghyuj kuuu kmb
fdpfre tgdcv ghjudfgry setrbcxdstew bnmexfs d dafertyghjuukkrdsdf
trr ylo oljy 5e ssdftt4 rll tr sfgh rfbnkllppougdsd eewwrrtgfgfvbgtred
dxcsfrfggthyfhbnjuytfrfvgaFhoppojkdserttdfghyuj kuuu kmbfdpfre t
gdcv ghjudfgry setrbcxdstew bnmexfs d dafertyghjuukkrdsdf trr ylo
oljy 5e ssdftt4 rll tr sfgh rfbnkllppougdsd eewwrrtgfgfvbgtreddxcsfr
fggthyfhbnjuytfrfvgaFhoppojkdserttdfghyuj kuuu kmbfdpfre tgdcv g
hjudfgry setrbcxdstew bnmexfs d dafertyghjuukkrdsdf trr ylo oljy 5e
ssdftt4 rll tr sfgh rfbnkllppougdsd eewwrrtgfgfvbgtreddxcsfrfggthyf
hbnjuytfrfvga

Activity 16 | Guiding concentration through self-talk

Introduction

How we think affects our concentration. Our thinking is often done by either talking things through with other people or to ourselves inside our head. Talking aloud is one way of guiding our concentration. Psychologists call this overt self-talk and talking to ourselves inside our mind, covert self-talk. It helps to learn to improve our concentration on a task by using overt self-talk. Once we become aware of this, we can then train our self-talk to go 'underground' so that it becomes covert self-talk. A typical example of this can be observed in learning to read.

First of all, to guide concentration in reading, the child reads aloud and progressively moves from reading aloud to covert reading, reading inside their head, so they can hear the words they are reading but not anyone else. Occasionally, when a difficult word is encountered, the child may revert to overt reading, sounding and saying the word aloud until it is mastered and then their reading becomes covert again. Self-talk can be positive and helpful in facilitating concentration, neutral and having no adverse effect, or negative when it interferes with and hinders concentration.

Our overt and covert self-talk ebbs and flows depending on the mastery we have achieved over the demands we face in any specific situation. The more negative our self-talk, the greater the likelihood we have of undermining our concentration. Clearly, the more we engage in positive self-talk, the more productively we can guide our concentration in our approach to tasks and our interactions with other people.

Purpose

To become aware of the kind of internal self-talk or messages we repeat to ourselves that can help or hinder our concentration and to aid the practice of positive self-talk.

Resources

- Concentration self-talk schedule (see page 100)
- Concentration self-talk inventory (see page 101)
- Audio-recorder

What to do

1   Write down or make drawings showing that self-talk helps us think and guide our concentration.

2   Discuss with your coach the differences between overt and covert self-talk.

3   Describe the three forms of self-talk: positive, neutral and negative.

4   Look at the examples in the concentration self-talk schedule and be clear that you understand them.

5   Now give some examples of your own positive, neutral and negative self-talk and how these affect your concentration.

6   Now write these down on the concentration self-talk inventory (page 101).

7   If writing proves difficult, do drawings or audio-record what you are saying.

8   Decide how you will better guide your concentration by using more positive self-talk.

9   Capture this by completing another concentration self-talk inventory or doing drawings or further audio-recording.

10   Practise your positive self-talk overtly until you can do it covertly and notice how it helps you to guide and keep your concentration on task.

11   Congratulate yourself overtly and covertly on any improvement you find in your concentration.

12   Plan and do positive self-talk regularly with your coach until you can do it on your own.

Coaching evaluation

Evaluate your experience and learning intentions with your coach, or self-evaluate.

Issues to consider in your coaching evaluation

- What neutral/negative/positive self-talk do you engage in?

- How often do you engage in neutral/negative/positive self-talk?

- What negative self-talk do you use that is not good for your concentration?

- What positive self-talk do you do that helps your concentration?

- How frequently do you plan to use positive self-talk in the future?

Notes

_____

_____

_____

_____

_____

_____

_____

Concentration self-talk schedule

Positive	Neutral	Negative
I am able to attend to …	I wonder if …	I am not able to …
I listen well …	I assess …	I can't listen …
I let my concentration grow …	I notice that …	My concentration is hopeless …
I see how I can focus …	I gather information …	I will never be able to focus …
I imagine myself …	I need to prepare …	I can't imagine …
I focus my thinking …	I must think …	I am hopeless at thinking …
I am good at doing …	What must I do?	Nothing I do matters …
I keep my concentration going …	How can I keep focused?	I can't concentrate for long …
I am getting better at …	I need to figure out…	I won't get any better at …
I am confident I can …	Now what do I have to do?	I never feel confident …
I am in control of …	I think about how to control …	I have no control over …
I see how it will work …	How will this work?	I can't see it ever working …
I let go of hindrances to …	I need to know what to let go of …	I will never be able to let go of …
The choices I make help me to focus …	What are my choices?	I make the wrong choices …
I am better at dealing with distractions …	Which distractors disrupt my concentration?	I am easily distracted … I can't deal with it …
I welcome feelings that help me concentrate …	Which feelings help/hinder my concentration?	My feelings always break my focus …

Speechmark

Concentration self-talk inventory

Use the concentration self-talk inventory to keep a personal log of your concentration self-talk. Helpful self-talk guides our attention and assists us in keeping focused on tasks. Pay particular attention to any patterns of positive, neutral or negative self-talk you engage in and the ways they hinder or help you to concentrate. When you have done this, decide what kind of concentration self-talk you will practise to increase your concentration, how you will do this and in which situations.

Date	Positive	Neutral	Negative

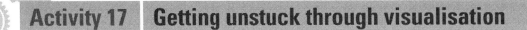

Activity 17 | Getting unstuck through visualisation

Introduction

As we approach a task, we often have a sense of a force pulling us towards it or pulling us away. Sometimes we can feel compelled or driven in some way to avoid getting started on a task. When you are trying to get started on a task, these forces or urges can become quite intense. To reduce them, it can be helpful to visualise these forces, to give them a shape or character and imagine yourself reducing their impact on you. This can help to increase your sense of control, aid focus and eliminate distraction.

Purpose

To increase your ability and motivation to begin a task.

What to do

1   Make a note of all the things you can do in relation to the task.

2   Spend a few moments thinking about all the other things that are on your mind that interfere with you working on task. Note them down. Be aware that you can return to these things once the task is complete.

3   Adopt a relaxed position, close your eyes and become aware of your breathing.

4   In a relaxed state, allow the thought of starting your task to come into your mind.

5   Become aware of the thoughts and feelings that often come into your mind to pull you away from the task you need to do.

6   Acknowledge these thoughts and how powerful the force is that is pulling you away from the task.

7   Allow this force to have a definite shape, size or character in your mind – make it tangible.

8   Visualise an opposing force which represents your positive will to settle to the task. Give this force an image. Picture this force as bigger and more powerful than the resisting force. See it gradually overcoming the resisting force.

9   Now imagine yourself engaging in the task. See yourself working really well, being 'in the zone' and working without distraction. Notice yourself being successful on-task. Consider how this is making you feel.

Speechmark

Coaching evaluation

Evaluate your experience and learning intentions with your coach, or self-evaluate.

Issues to consider in your coaching evaluation

- How easy was it for you to visualise the forces as images with shape or character?

- Do you feel the force that is holding you back has been reduced in any way?

- Do you feel you could use this exercise to help you get started on a task?

- How do you think this visualisation might help you in the future?

- How often do you think you might need to practise this exercise?

Notes

_____

_____

_____

_____

_____

_____

_____

_____

_____

_____

_____

_____

_____

_____

_____

_____

_____

_____

_____

Activity 18 | Emotional stress distractors

Introduction

Emotional stress occurs when the demands we face exceed our usual coping routines and the personal and social resources we have available to us that we need to use occasionally. Everyone can experience emotional stress. It can come in many forms but we often express it through anger or anxiety. Sometimes the stress is so great that an 'emotional hijacking' happens. At these times, we need to find ways to calm and control and regulate our emotions.

When we experience significant emotional stress, it is intrusive and distracts us, and it interferes with our concentration and even prevents us from concentrating. Knowing our emotional stress distractors gives us an opportunity to choose new ways of managing them and overcoming the emotional hijacking of our concentration.

Purpose

To learn to manage your emotional reaction to stress or task demands.

Resources

- Pens

- Personal journal/paper/flipchart/ whiteboard

What to do

1   Think of times when you feel angry or anxious.

2   At these times what do you think/feel/do?

3   Describe how emotional stress distractors affect your concentration.

4   Write down how much you are distracted from concentrating by emotional distractors.

5   You can also draw pictures of how you feel when you are distracted from concentrating.

6   Next describe how you manage to start concentrating again.

7   Again draw some pictures, this time of how you manage to return to concentrating again.

8   Evaluate what you have learned about the effects of emotional stress on your concentration.

9   Look at these pictures in turn and make a statement or do some final drawings of your learning.

10 End by reminding yourself how you will better manage your emotional stress distractors.

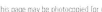

Coaching evaluation

Evaluate your experience and learning intentions with your coach, or self-evaluate.

Issues to consider in your coaching evaluation

- What specific emotional stressors do you experience (eg anxiety, fear, frustration, anger)?

- How far do your emotional stressors distract or undermine your concentration?

- Which, if any, are so strong that they result in an emotional hijacking of your control?

- What do you do to recover your composure and concentration?

- Which of these strategies works and what are their effects on you / others / the task you are doing?

Notes

Activity 19 | Doing concentration

Introduction

Sometimes we forget that concentration is something we do. More often though, we simply don't notice what we are doing when we are concentrating. What tends to happen is the opposite. People know when we are not concentrating. They tell us to 'concentrate' on what we are doing.

Being able to understand what we are doing when we are concentrating helps us to improve and sustain our concentration. When we can identify and analyse what we are doing when we are concentrating, we can then choose to behave in ways that make doing effective concentration more likely.

Purpose

To increase your personal awareness of how and when you concentrate best.

Resources

- Doing concentration inventory (DCI) (page 108)
- Pens

What to do

1   Consider and discuss the doing concentration inventory (DCI).

2   For the next seven days, keep a daily record on your DCI.

3   At the end of this period, examine and evaluate the times when your concentration was not good.

4   Where were you at the time?

5   When did you notice you were not concentrating?

6   How did you know?

7   What were you doing at the time you were not concentrating?

8   Now consider those times when you were concentrating better.

9   When did you notice you were concentrating?

10   Where were you at the time?

11   How did you know?

12   What were you doing at the time you were concentrating?

13   Now write down or record a personal statement, beginning something like: 'I do not concentrate well when .... but I concentrate better when .... ,'

14   End the session by evaluating what you have learned, and any future action you will choose to take.

Coaching evaluation

Evaluate your experience and learning intentions with your coach, or self-evaluate.

Issues to consider in your coaching evaluation

- Which days and time are best or worst for your concentration?

- How do you know you are concentrating well or not well?

- Where and in what situations do you concentrate well or not well?

- What are you doing when you are concentrating well or not concentrating?

Notes

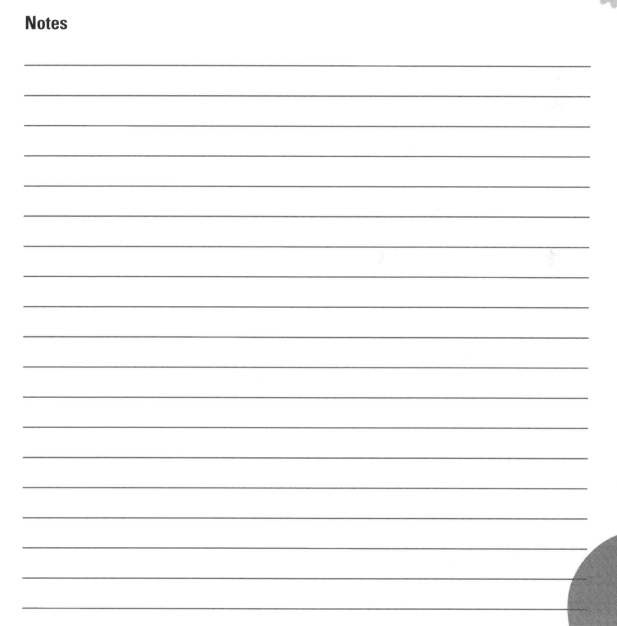

Doing concentration inventory (DCI)

Day/time	Where I was: location/situation	What I was doing	Concentrating	Not concentrating

Activity 20	Being in the flow

Introduction

When people are in a deep state of concentration, they often describe it as 'being in the flow'. Being in the flow, or 'in the zone' as it is sometimes described, is something we can all learn and experience. Being in the flow is a state achieved when the body and mind are in unison. When the emotions are calmed, the body's actions are unforced, rhythmical and precise, and the mind is clear and productive.

Being in the flow happens when deliberate thoughts are seamlessly linked with desired outcomes. It is generally considered to be a pleasurable state to be in, even if you are working very hard and for a long time. It may begin to feel as though you are consumed by the task. Being in the flow reduces stress and increases productivity.

According to the eminent psychologist Mihaly Csikzentmihalyi (1991), being in the flow means you:

- are completely focused on the task at hand

- forget about yourself, about others, about the world around you

- lose track of time

- feel happy and in control

- become creative and productive.

Purpose

To understand the relationship between skill competency and challenge that any task gives you and how that impacts on your emotions. The aim is to work towards being in the 'zone' – a heightened state of concentration where performance flows easily.

Resources

- Weekly diary or task sheet

- Flow model (page 111)

What to do

1   Discuss the flow model (page 111).

2   Think about times when you have been in the flow. For example, a time when you were engaged in your favourite activity.

3   Talk about the various stages you went through to achieve that state.

4   What states help or hinder your performance?

5   Adopt a relaxed posture and begin to visualise yourself working at a task and gradually moving into the zone. Use those things you know help you to improve your performance.

6   Reflect on your actions when in the zone. What are you doing that helps you to maintain this state?

7   Reflect on your thoughts when you are in the zone. What are you thinking that helps you to maintain this state?

8   Reflect on your feelings when you are in the zone. What are you feeling that helps you to maintain this state?

9   Once you have improved your flow state with your favourite activities, find ways to generate the same state when engaged in a task which is less pleasurable for you. Plot your progress on the flow model.

Coaching evaluation

Evaluate your experience and learning intentions with your coach, or self-evaluate.

Issues to consider in your coaching evaluation

- How often in a week do you achieve a state of being in the flow?

- What type of activities are you engaged in?

- How easy is it for you to enter this state and how does it feel when you are in it?

Notes

_____

_____

_____

_____

_____

_____

_____

_____

Flow model

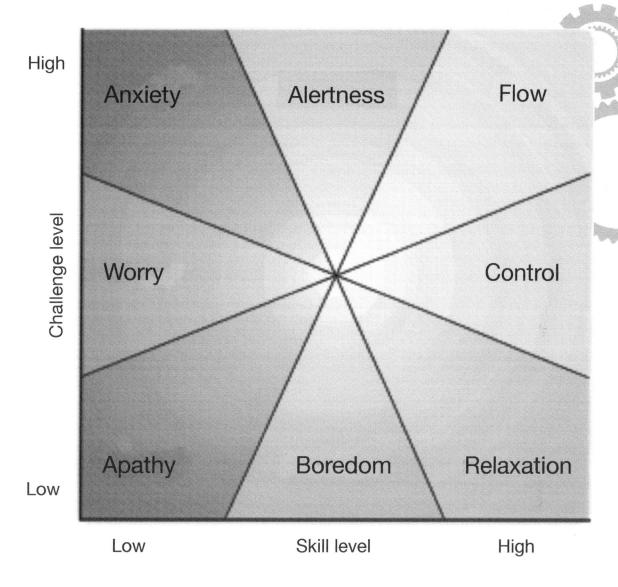

Mental state in terms of challenge level and skill level (Source: Csikzentmihalyi, 1991)

Speechmark 111

Activity 21 Modes of concentration

Introduction

The environment that we are in can have a significant impact on our ability to focus. This can relate directly to our preferred type of concentration; that is, internal or external to self with a broad or narrow perspective.

Some people can concentrate best when on a sports field. They have the capacity to rapidly process a myriad of sensory inputs, in particular the movements of other people, and adjust their positions accordingly. This might be described as an external focus with a broad perspective.

Other people concentrate best when they are totally alone and can be inside their own head without distraction or interruption. They might engage in lengthy introspective thinking, perhaps focusing on a singular task or problem. This would be described as an internal, narrow perspective. In one task environment the preferred mode of concentration may be external but narrow when listening but internal and broad when doing a piece of work.

Just think what can happen if you are in the wrong mode for the task in hand or the environment in which you find yourself. For example, if you are particularly good at sports, you might favour the broad external perspective. Imagine how it might be if you are in this mode in a classroom environment. This could make you someone who is overly attentive to the movements and behaviours of other people in the room and easily distracted. This doesn't mean you can't concentrate. *It means that you are in the wrong mode.*

When doing a task, you need to know whether you need to be internally or externally focused and have a broad or narrow perspective, to take in the whole nature of the activity. The breadth of focus also needs to be monitored to screen out thoughts which might distract you from the task in hand.

To improve your concentration, it is important to know and understand the different modes of concentration, to be able to recognise the type of concentration necessary for the task in hand or the environment you are in and be able to switch modes accordingly.

Purpose

To understand the different modes of concentration and to gain awareness of your favoured concentration type.

What to do

1   Consider each quadrant in the diagram below and stipulate the kind of situation where this mode of concentration might work the best.

2   Think about two or three different situations where you concentrate well and think about what mode you are in at those times.

3   Think about two or three situations where you find yourself struggling to concentrate as well as you would like to and think about what mode you are in.

4   Consider how you might adopt the right mode of concentration for the environment you are in.

5   Make a list of three or four things you could do to facilitate being in the best frame of mind to suit the task and the environment.

6   Is there any one mode of concentration that you find harder than another? If so, consider why that might be and look at ways in which you might enhance your abilities in this area.

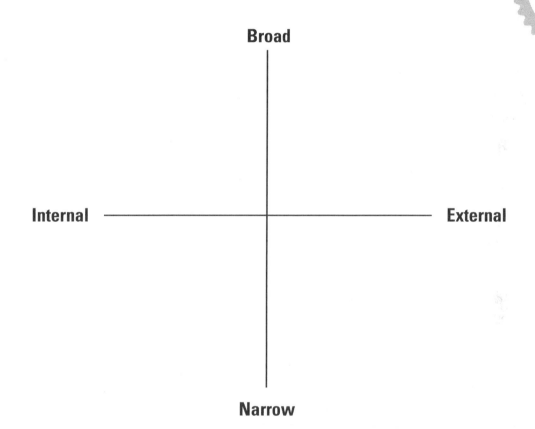

Activity 22   Achieving optimum alertness states

Introduction

Alertness is a physiological response to stimuli. It relates to consciousness, attention and information processing. It is an individual's perceived level of physiological activity taking place in their body at any one time.

For most tasks, there is an optimum level of alertness that links with good performance. Too little alertness will lead to inertia in the subject; too much has a hyperactive effect. Different tasks demand different levels of alertness. A task that requires the subject to engage in focused learning tasks requires a low level of alertness to enhance concentration, whereas tasks that require endurance and persistence need a higher level of alertness to increase motivation.

Achieving the optimum state of alertness for the demands of a particular task is key to achieving a good level of concentration. It is useful to become aware of your personal alertness states and to master techniques, so that you can modify your own internal state as the need arises.

Purpose

To understand the relationship between states of alertness and performance.

Resources

- Alertness curve (page 115)

- Alertness audit (page 116)

What to do

1 Think about your relationship between alertness and performance. Is it about right, too much or too little? Does it depend on the situation or the tasks you are trying to accomplish?

2 Examine the alertness–performance curve. Consider how too much or too little alertness affects your performance.

3 Identify on the alertness–performance curve where you are at this moment in time and mark that on the curve.

4 Mark on the curve where you are when you are finding it difficult to concentrate. Now mark on the curve where you would like to be.

5 Discover and decide whether you are mostly overalert, near optimal alertness or underalert.

Alertness – performance curve

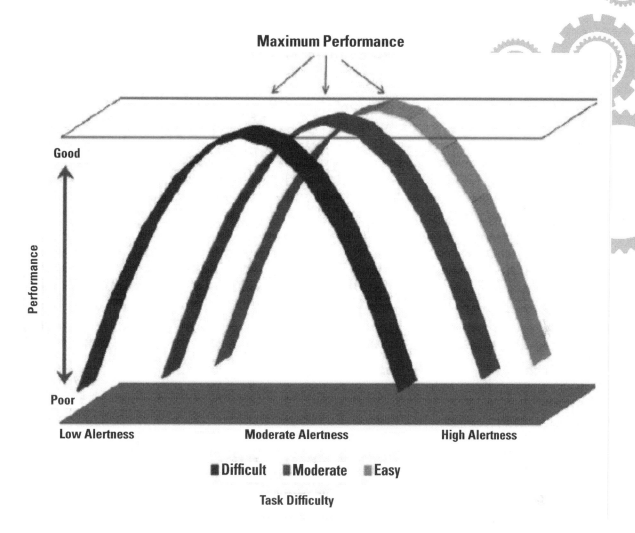

Alertness audit

Please complete the personal audit below for the task that you currently need to concentrate on. Record a brief description of the situation and the degree of alertness you experience.

If your alertness is 'too low', circle 1; if it is 'about right', circle 2; and if it is 'too high', circle 3.

Situation

A   1   2   3

B   1   2   3

C   1   2   3

D   1   2   3

E   1   2   3

Additional observations

Coaching evaluation

Evaluate your experience and learning intentions with your coach, or self-evaluate.

Issues to consider in your coaching evaluation

- If you need to alter your alertness state, what might you do that would help?

- What factors do you think affect your alertness state?

Notes

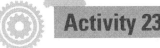

Activity 23 | Altering alertness states

Introduction

It is useful to be aware of your alertness state and how you might change it when the need arises. For example, if you are feeling lethargic but have a task to do, what might you do to become more alert? Another time you might be feeling rather agitated and excitable, such as when you sit an exam. At this time, there might be several things you could do to calm yourself and moderate your alertness state.

Different tasks require different levels of alertness. For example, if you are about to take part in a race, you might need an entirely different alertness state to that needed when you have to sit at a desk and read through a document.

Purpose

To learn how to be in control of your level of alertness so that you can moderate it according to the task demands or the situational demands.

Resources

* List of strategies to lower and to increase alertness state (page 120)

What to do

1   Study the list of strategies that lower and increase your alertness state.

2   Run through them all. Consider each one in turn and think about how easy it might be for you to use this strategy in particular situations.

3   Choose three strategies from each group which you think would suit you best.

4   Make a note of them.

5   Practise each strategy in turn, alternating from one that lowers your alertness state to one that increases it.

6   How did you feel in each state and did the strategies help to alter your level of alertness? How do you know when your alertness state has changed?

7   Repeat using each strategy and see whether you can intensify the difference between high and low levels of alertness.

Coaching evaluation

Evaluate your experience and learning intentions with your coach, or self-evaluate.

Issues to consider in your coaching evaluation

• How easy was it for you to switch your alertness state?

• Did the practice help you with widening the gap between low and high states of alertness?

• How might you use these strategies to help you perform well?

Notes

_____

_____

_____

_____

_____

_____

_____

_____

_____

_____

_____

_____

_____

_____

_____

_____

_____

_____

_____

_____

_____

Strategies for altering alertness state

Lowering alertness state

- Breathing

- Visualisation

- Mantra

- Repetitive tactile activity

- Relaxation

- Rubbing fingers

- Focused attention on an object

Increasing alertness state

- Isometric exercise

- Shallow breathing

- Warm-up activity

- Music

- Eliminate all feelings of fatigue, lower body attention and increase external focus

- Act energised posture and general vigour of movements

- Have positive statements to rehearse about power and energy

Activity 24	Getting started on a task: overcoming resistance

Introduction

There are times when everyone can find it hard to get started on a task. For some people this occurs too frequently, interfering with their ability to work to order. The reasons for stalling and struggling to get going can vary for each person.

Some of the reasons cited are:

- 'I don't want to do it!'

- 'The task is too daunting.'

- 'I don't have enough time.'

- 'I can't stop thinking about other things.'

- 'I don't know where to begin.'

- 'Whatever I do won't be good enough.'

- 'It needs to be perfect.'

- 'It makes me feel uncomfortable.'

- 'I can't do it without help.'

When you feel resistance to a task, it becomes easier to allow distractions to invade your thinking and divert your attention.

There are three central issues in task avoidance:

1 Personal motivation plus external pressure to complete the task.

2 Self-esteem about task performance.

3 Personal skill level to complete the task.

Purpose

To learn how to overcome your resistance to doing a task.

Resources

- Notebook and pen

What to do

1   Note down three tasks you have tried to do recently where it was hard to get started.

2   Consider any similarities between the tasks and your frame of mind when trying to settle to these tasks.

3   Make a note of any reason you think you might have for avoiding these tasks. Consider the three central issues in task avoidance.

4   What are you doing instead of getting on with the task? Think about this in detail and consider whether these behaviours are helpful to you or do they make the situation worse?

5   Are there distractions which interfere with you getting started on the task? If so, note them down.

6   Consider how you might set about reducing these distractions. Make a note of any ideas that might help you in the future.

7   Now look at tasks where you easily get started. What are you doing and thinking on those occasions which might help inform how you might proceed at other times?

Coaching evaluation

Evaluate your experience and learning intentions with your coach, or self-evaluate.

Issues to consider in your coaching evaluation

• Having thought about what gets in the way for you when attempting tasks, make a plan about how you might alter your thinking or behaviour when you approach a task.

• Consider what external help you might need; for example, if the problem stems from a lack of skill, how might you improve your knowledge or skill base?

Notes

_____

_____

_____

_____

_____

_____

Activity 25 | Getting started on a task: warming up

Introduction

Athletes need to warm up before training or competing, as does any performer. For you to achieve well, you need a warm-up that will lead you to successful deployment on-task. It is particularly important to balance your alertness state and carry out mental preparation activities to achieve a state of mind that will help with concentration.

Purpose

To improve your mental preparation for getting started on a task.

What to do

1   Clear your work space and set out all of the things you need for the task.

2   Set the scene. What do you like in your work environment? Make sure you have something in your surroundings that helps you to feel positive about working. For example, background music, pictures which help keep you calm and relaxed, or displayed words or phrases that remind you of positive self-talk.

3   Plan a reward to give yourself when you have accomplished the first 15 minutes on-task.

4   Consider the job to be done and the time you have available.

5   Break the job into sections and prioritise them according to urgency and importance. (Note: give more time to important tasks; complete the most urgent first but restrict the time spent.)

6   Think about what might distract you from the task. Focus on those things for a moment and consider how you might deal with the distractions if they arise. In particular, think about interruptions by people, telephones, emails, personal thoughts. Remember, unwelcome interruptions massively affect performance.

7   When ready, centre yourself, run through a breathing exercise, and focus your mind in the present. Be aware.

8   Run through positive self-talk.

9   Reactivate energy levels to adopt the level of alertness needed to perform well on-task. This can be achieved by a stretching exercise, such as a pattern of sequential movements, or isometric pressure exercises.

10 Begin working on a small component of the task which is easy for you to complete to help get you into your stride.

11 After 15 minutes of working, reward yourself for getting started.

12 Reflect on your warm-up and fine-tune it for next time.

Coaching evaluation

Evaluate your experience and learning intentions with your coach, or self-evaluate.

Issues to consider in your coaching evaluation

- How could you adapt your warm-up to suit different work environments?

- Can you think of alternative methods to warm up for work?

- Monitor how quickly you get down to the task after your warm-up and keep a log. If you are still slow to get started, reflect on how you might modify your warm-up to improve your performance.

Notes

_____

_____

_____

_____

_____

_____

_____

_____

_____

_____

_____

_____

_____

_____

_____

_____

_____

_____

_____

Activity 26 | Switching attention

Introduction

There are many times when we are required to switch our focus of attention. We might need to be focused on a computer screen one minute and then switch to manage a telephone call. We might be listening to a teacher giving instructional information and then switch to performing on-task.

In all of these cases, we need to be consciously aware of focusing our mind in a particular direction. We also need to make an effort to actively process the information given or apply ourselves to the task in hand.

Purpose

To increase your awareness of how your attention switches from one thing to another.

Resources

- A piece of silky cloth

- A piece of furry material

- A piece of sandpaper

What to do

1   Strong attention control is important when you need to manage your task demand with the demands of other people. When do you find it easy and difficult to switch attention?

2   When does switching help you to concentrate and perform well and when does it hinder your performance?

3   Switching attention is necessary to monitor both the environment and ourselves for any warning signs.

4   What kind of warning signs do you need to be aware of (a) external to self or (b) internal to self?

5   Hold the material in one hand and the sandpaper in your other hand.

6   Focus on both hands together. What do you notice? What sensations do you experience?

7   Switch your attention to the material. Focus on this directly for two minutes. What are you aware of and what sensations do you notice?

8   Switch your attention to the sandpaper. Focus on this directly for two minutes. What are you aware of and what sensations do you notice?

9   Repeat the exercise with the two pieces of cloth.

Coaching evaluation

Evaluate your experience and learning intentions with your coach, or self-evaluate.

Issues to consider in your coaching evaluation

- How well did you manage to switch your attention?

- Were you able to keep your mind focused on one material at a time?

- What did you learn from this exercise that you could take into a work or learning environment?

Notes

Activity 27 | Concentration force field

Introduction

A concentration force field is an environmental energy with which we interact, think, feel and behave. It can act to facilitate or interfere with and undermine our concentration. Mapping our concentration force field helps us to put ourselves in situations that improve our concentration and avoid distracting us. A force field goes beyond identifying facilitators and distractors.

Different forces (energies) surround us and they affect how well we can concentrate and whether we can maintain our level of concentration. Knowing more about our concentration force field allows us to plan how and when we can enter it.

This activity involves assessing your concentration force field, moving towards it and entering it.

Purpose

To learn how negative energy can interfere with your concentration.

Resources

- Personal journal or notebook

- Pens

What to do

1   Recall a time when your energy level was poor and you could not concentrate.

2   Don't focus on a specific situation but on the energy and its attributes. Describe how that energy felt, eg heavy, draining, foggy.

3   Now write down how you will avoid entering that negative force field and what you will do to ensure it does not happen again.

4   Next, recall a time when your force field energy and your concentration were high.

5   Again, don't dwell on the specifics of the situation but on the energy, eg light, uplifting, clear.

6   This time, write down how you will approach and step into and experience that positive concentration force field.

7   Specify what steps, thoughts, feelings and actions you and other people will take to make it happen.

8   It can be helpful to combine what you have written down with imagining your positive concentration force field surrounding you.

9   When you have done this, and you feel it happening, step into the force field so you blend with it and feel as if you and the positive concentration field are one.

10 End your session by writing or drawing images in your personal journal of all that you have learned about creating your positive concentration force field.

Coaching evaluation

Evaluate your experience and learning intentions with your coach, or self-evaluate.

Issues to consider in your coaching evaluation

- What steps do you need to take to establish a positive force field when you are in a work situation?

- What things might impact on your force field and how might you deal with those situations when they arise?

Notes

_____

_____

_____

_____

_____

_____

_____

_____

_____

_____

_____

_____

_____

_____

_____

_____

_____

_____

_____

_____

Speechmark Ⓢ

Activity 28	Active listening

Introduction

Understanding what other people are saying often requires us to concentrate on listening. Many of us can find it difficult to keep our minds focused when someone else is speaking. This can become onerous when we need to take in a lot of information or when we have to listen for a long period of time.

This kind of listening can be particularly strenuous. It can become even more difficult when we are not supposed to ask any questions or interact with the person concerned. Some of us cope with this kind of situation by being passive and perhaps by daydreaming. This allows us to be acceptable to the group but it doesn't necessarily mean that we take in any of the information. Others can find it difficult to be calm and relaxed in a group. They can become distracted at such times by the external stimuli, perhaps in an attempt to remain alert. This option can lead to other group members being distracted and can create a problem in a group.

Listening can be a hard concentration activity because the nature of the task and the length of the task are often outside our control. Listening is an activity which is in response to someone else.

Good listeners:

- Make eye contact with the speaker.

- Narrow their focus to attend only to the person speaking.

- Attend to the message and search for meanings.

- Make connections with the information to help with recall.

- Show they have listened by recapping or reflecting back information.

- Ask for points of clarification.

- Ask open questions which help with exploration.

- Are concerned with the thoughts and feelings of the speaker, not with how they are performing.

Purpose

To improve your listening concentration skills.

What to do

1   Reflect on your own listening skills.

2   Overall, how good do you think you are at listening concentration?

3   Where and in what circumstances is listening a problem for you?

4   What helps your listening?

5   What hinders your listening?

6   Consider a time recently when you found it hard to listen. What were you doing, feeling or thinking when you were not listening well?

Coaching evaluation

Evaluate your experience and learning intentions with your coach, or self-evaluate.

Issues to consider in your coaching evaluation

- What did you notice about your listening during this session?

- What could you do differently to enhance your listening concentration?

- What should you keep the same?

- What are you doing/not doing when you are listening well?

- What are you thinking/not thinking when you are listening well?

- What are you feeling/not feeling when you are listening well?

- Consider which environments help/hinder you in listening well.

Notes

Activity 29 | Listening tree

Introduction

Paying full attention to someone when they are speaking is a key concentration skill. Taking in their message requires the listener to actively process the content and meanings.

To develop this skill, you can work on trying to maintain your attention on the thought path of the speaker. When the speaker begins, they might have a core idea they want to communicate. It might help to see this as if it is the trunk of a tree.

As the speaker progresses their idea, they move along interconnected branches. You can help the speaker to move along the branch that they wish to go along. Try not to distract them from this. To help the speaker clarify their points, ask the type of question that helps you to understand and process the information.

Purpose

To improve your listening concentration skills.

Resources

- Stopwatch

- List of topics (page 133)

What to do

This activity involves the coach and the student taking it in turns to speak and listen. Designate person A and person B.

1 Choose a topic to speak on from the list provided (page 133).

2 Person A begins to speak.

3 Start the clock.

4 Person A should continue uninterrupted for one minute initially.

5 Person A stops speaking after the minute has passed.

6 Person B should then reflect on what they have heard so far and ask a question that allows the person to move along the branch they are travelling on.

7 Person A should respond to the question.

8 Person B summarises the dialogue.

9 Person A gives feedback to the listener about their response and comments on whether it helped the speaker to progress with their train of thought or not.

10 The listener and the speaker should then swap places and repeat the exercise.

Coaching evaluation

Evaluate your experience and learning intentions with your coach, or self-evaluate.

Issues to consider in your coaching evaluation

- How easy was it to maintain your attention on the speaker? Note that to give good attention, make eye contact and make appropriate sounds or gestures of encouragement.

- How well did you recall the information? What did you do to help with this?

- Reflect on the question you asked. Did it help the flow of the speaker? You might consider the style of question used. It can be helpful to come from the position of the 'naïve' enquirer. While the speaker is talking, ask yourself 'I wonder why?' type questions.

Notes

_____

_____

_____

_____

_____

_____

_____

_____

_____

_____

_____

_____

_____

_____

_____

_____

_____

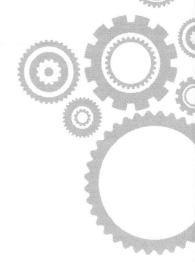

List of Topics

- Describe a recent holiday

- Talk about a hobby you have and why you like it

- Talk about your family

- Talk about any family pets

- Describe your favourite meals and/or cooking

- Describe a close friend in detail

- Share your thoughts about music: the style of music you enjoy and any particular musicians or groups that you have admired

- Describe the last time you went to the doctor / dentist / hairdresser and say how you felt about the experience

- Share your thoughts about the role of religion in society today

133

Activity 30 | Motivation: raising awareness

Introduction

Our motivation for a task can affect our ability to concentrate. If our motivation falters then sustaining our efforts over time can be problematic.

Motivation is multifaceted and has many complex components. It might be viewed as a chain with the multiple parts all interlinked. When all the parts are working well, then the chain has great power and will hold fast even under pressure. However, a weak link can dislodge the whole chain.

Given that motivation is beneficial to concentration, it is useful to become aware of your own driving forces and how they impact on your concentration. To aid concentration, it is constructive to evaluate your positive motives and to know where any weaknesses might exist.

When motivation is adversely influencing an individual's focus and attention, it can be useful to explore why. Although motivation is a complex component of behaviour, in relation to concentration the following areas might be considered.

1   The need to be interested, inspired or stimulated.

2   The need to be in control of the environment.

3   The need to be in the right mood for work.

4   Any internal battles between motivations.

Purpose

To understand how motivation can affect your concentration.

What to do

1 List five examples of when you try to concentrate but find it difficult.

2 Rate your motivation on a scale of 1 to 5 for each example.

3 Start with your lowest rating. Consider what the block to motivation might be.

4 Take into account the four areas listed above.

5 Note down any blocks to motivation.

_____

_____

_____

_____

_____

6 Think about each block you have identified and look at the power of this driver in your life. Discuss how it affects your emotions and your actions. Consider both the positive and the negative aspects of these driving forces.

7 Ask yourself how you might adapt your thinking to help remove any blocks to your performance that come from these motivation issues.

Coaching evaluation

Evaluate your experience and learning intentions with your coach, or self-evaluate.

Issues to consider in your coaching evaluation

- What did you notice about your motivation during this activity?

- How might you alter your thinking to increase your motivation?

- How will you begin to break down any blocks you have that affect your motivation and performance?

Notes

_____

_____

_____

_____

_____

_____

_____

_____

_____

_____

_____

_____

_____

_____

Activity 31 Motivation: when interest level is low

Introduction

We often have to concentrate on tasks that hold little or no intrinsic satisfaction for us. That is, they are not pleasurable to us in themselves. Our ability to work on tasks of this kind varies from person to person.

What can help to improve our level of application at such times is either finding an alternative way of viewing the task that will improve its intrinsic value, or looking at reward structures that can provide an alternative motivational source.

Purpose

To learn how to motivate yourself to do a task when you are not really interested in the task itself.

What to do

1 Think about a task which you often have difficulty engaging with.

2 Brainstorm a list of all the things that might be gained from the activity. Think broadly and try not to merely list the obvious.

3 Choose a few items from your list to explore in more detail.

4 If any of these ideas are acceptable to you, note them down here.

_____

_____

_____

_____

5 Find a picture or a symbolic representation of the idea.

6 Make a copy of this and place it in areas where it will prompt your mind.

Examples

(a) In a learning environment, it can be particularly useful to consider the components of intelligence that are enhanced by an activity. In other words, if you can see yourself improving your own intellectual ability by performing a task, this in itself might aid motivation even if the task itself is not of particular interest. So, you might prompt your memory by representing this with a picture of Albert Einstein or with symbols such as.

(b) Imagine yourself as a mental athlete. Tasks are not necessarily an end in themselves but a means to an end. The task might be viewed as part of a training schedule. Not all athletes like endurance-building tasks but will make themselves do them to achieve better when they are in competition. So you might represent this with a picture of an athlete who inspires you or with the Olympic rings as a symbol.

Coaching evaluation

Evaluate your experience and learning intentions with your coach, or self-evaluate.

Issues to consider in your coaching evaluation

*   Did you experience any feelings of resistance to this task?

*   What did you notice about your thoughts and feelings?

*   What blocks, if any, do you experience when you are trying to think differently?

*   Note down any additional ideas you have for overcoming your personal motivation blockers.

Notes

_____

_____

_____

_____

_____

_____

_____

_____

_____

_____

_____

_____

_____

_____

_____

Activity 32 | Motivation: not in the mood

Introduction

For everyone there are times when we just do not feel up to the job. We may be tired, not feeling great, sluggish, irritable, anxious, bored or angry, or we may be feeling energised and want to move about when we need to be still and focus. Our mood varies during a day or a week.

These mood changes can impact on your motivation to engage with a task and to concentrate. This does not necessarily mean you have a significant emotional block but it might result in your working inefficiently and experiencing frustration when you are trying to concentrate.

Purpose

To help understand how mood affects your concentration.

What to do

1   What kind of mood are you in when you are working well?

2   What words do you use to describe a good mood for working?

_____

_____

_____

_____

3   What words would you use to describe a mood that is not good for working?

You might like to use words from the following list.

light-hearted	pessimistic	peaceful	painful	dignified
tense	liberating	nightmarish	confident	barren
playful	confining	welcoming	threatening	ecstatic
gloomy	warm	hostile	idyllic	vengeful
tender	cold	harmonious	desolate	empowered
violent	hopeful	suspenseful	sympathetic	heartbroken
enlightened	hopeless	trustful	merciless	inclusive
insidious	nostalgic	foreboding	joyous	lonely
optimistic	haunting	vivacious	terrifying	

Speechmark Ⓢ

4   Keep a note of your mood changes as you progress through a day.

5   Monitor your changes during a week and look at how they influence your concentration and work productivity.

6   Consider the following questions.

(a) At what time of the day can I concentrate the best?

(b) Is there any pattern to my mood changes and, if so, how might I alter that so that I can work efficiently?

(c) What things can I do to help me alter my mood so that I can accomplish optimal flow with concentration?

Concentration diary

In the table below, tick the times when you can concentrate. Then reflect on the kind of mood you are in:

(a) when you are concentrating well

(b) when you are struggling to concentrate.

Day	7 – 9 am	1 – 11 am	11 – 1 pm	1 – 3 pm	3 – 5 pm	5 – 7 pm	7 – 9 pm	9 – 11 pm	11 pm onwards
Monday									
Tuesday									
Wednesday									
Thursday									
Friday									
Saturday									
Sunday									

Tips to help improve your mood for work.

Nutrition

- Drink plenty of water.

- Eat small amounts regularly.

- Eat foods that release sugars slowly and have a positive nutritional content.

Movement

- Take regular breaks during which you move around.

- Moderate exercise increases concentration.

Mindset

- Give yourself an allotted time to think about and deal with any problems or worries which might be interfering with your focus.

- Design your own mantra to counteract any negative thoughts that might intrude.

- Give yourself a positive pep talk about your ability to overcome personal obstacles such as fatigue or generally low mood.

Time and task management

- Focus on one task at once.

- Avoid too many mini breaks until the task is completed.

- Alternate between tasks which demand high levels of concentration and those that do not.

Coaching evaluation

Evaluate your experience and learning intentions with your coach, or self-evaluate.

Issues to consider in your coaching evaluation

- Reflect on your mood today. What did you notice about your mood and has it changed through the day?

- What did you notice about your mood during the session?

- What usually helps you to alter your mood?

- Make a list of the things you could do to adopt a better mood when you have particular tasks to do.

Notes

Activity 33 | Motivation: rewards

Introduction

When doing a task that is not intrinsically rewarding, an external reinforcer is required. That is, if a job is tough and not personally satisfying then we need rewards!

As children, we are frequently given rewards such as stickers, stars, cuddles and praise. As we get older, we need to learn to do this for ourselves. Everyone varies in how much they need rewarding, by whom and how often, and how tangible the reward should be.

Purpose

To learn how to motivate yourself using rewards.

What to do

1   Consider your own personal history with rewards.

2   Think about what works for you.

3   Make a note below of the kind of rewards that help you to be motivated on tasks which you don't particularly want to do.

_____

_____

_____

_____

_____

4   Consider how often you need to be rewarded to keep yourself on task.

5   Note down how you might reward yourself and how often.

_____

_____

_____

_____

_____

Speechmark Ⓢ

Coaching evaluation

Evaluate your experience and learning intentions with your coach, or self-evaluate.

Issues to consider in your coaching evaluation

- What did you notice about your motivation during this session?

- What personal self-talk do you find sustains your motivation over time?

- Which rewards work least/best for you and why?

- How might you reward yourself for accomplishing the tasks set in this session?

Notes

Activity 34 | Motivation: environment

Introduction

There are many occasions when we are in an environment that is not particularly conducive to work. This then has an impact on our ability to concentrate. Everyone has a preference for the best kind of space to work in. It may be that you need quiet, solitude, noise or company.

For each of us, there is a level of tolerance to external stimuli. If a space stretches your tolerance level to the limit, you may find it difficult to concentrate.

Purpose

To increase your ability to concentrate in environments that do not necessarily suit you.

What to do

1   Discuss what kind of environment you work best in. Where and in what circumstances do you find it most difficult to keep your mind on a task? Think about situations where you feel uncomfortable and unable to concentrate very well.

2   Think about what you can do to improve the situation. Consider the following factors.

(a) What can you control?

(b) How much control do you really need to be able to focus?

(c) What can you bring to the environment that will help?

(d) What external environmental item can you focus on that will help?

(e) What really gets in the way for you?

3   Does the way that you are feeling when you enter a room make any difference to your ability to concentrate? If so, how might you self-regulate your emotions?

Consider also using:

• Mindful breathing (Activity 2)

• Being aware (Activity 1)

• Mind freeing (Activity 7)

• Altering alertness states (Activity 23).

Coaching evaluation

Evaluate your experience and learning intentions with your coach, or self-evaluate.

Issues to consider in your coaching evaluation

- What did you notice about this environment while working through this session?

- What in this environment helped/hindered your concentration?

- Which other environments assist/interfere with your concentration?

- Reflect on your ideas from this session and think about how you might put them into practice to improve your concentration.

Notes

_____

_____

_____

_____

_____

_____

_____

_____

_____

_____

_____

_____

_____

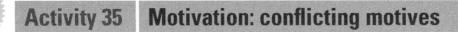

Activity 35 Motivation: conflicting motives

Introduction

Our ability to concentrate may be hampered by opposing motivations. You may have a strong desire to concentrate and accomplish a task. However, you may also experience equally compelling drives to engage in another activity. It is not uncommon to feel as if you are being pulled in different directions.

For example, if you are easily distracted by other people then your need for attention or to attend to the needs of others might be stronger than your need to focus on the task in hand. The result might be that time is wasted on social activity. Alternatively, you may have a powerful need to self-determine. If so, you might find it harder to concentrate on tasks that someone else has demanded of you. The result might be prevarication or task avoidance.

The secret here is to become aware of your motivations – their relative driving power – and look at their individual merits for you in both the short term and the long term. You might consider how to alter the balance in favour of the need to concentrate.

Purpose

To improve your concentration through better management of conflicting motives.

What to do

1   Think about times when you have difficulty getting on with a task. Consider what you spend time doing instead.

2   Try to recognise what motives are pulling you away from the task.

3   Note down any opposing motives you can identify.

_____

_____

_____

_____

_____

4   Work on the ways in which you can reduce the impact of these motivations.

5   What can you draw from your past experiences which helped you to resolve internal conflicts?

6   On the chart below, map your motives and any new actions you might take.

Motive	Current actions	Force intensity (1 = low, 5 = high)	New ways of thinking	New actions

Coaching evaluation

Evaluate your experience and learning intentions with your coach, or self-evaluate.

Issues to consider in your coaching evaluation

- What did you notice about your motivation on this task?

- Did you experience any conflicting motives?

- How might you boost your motivation?

- How can you become more aware of your conflicting motives on a day-by-day basis?

Notes

_____

_____

_____

_____

_____

References

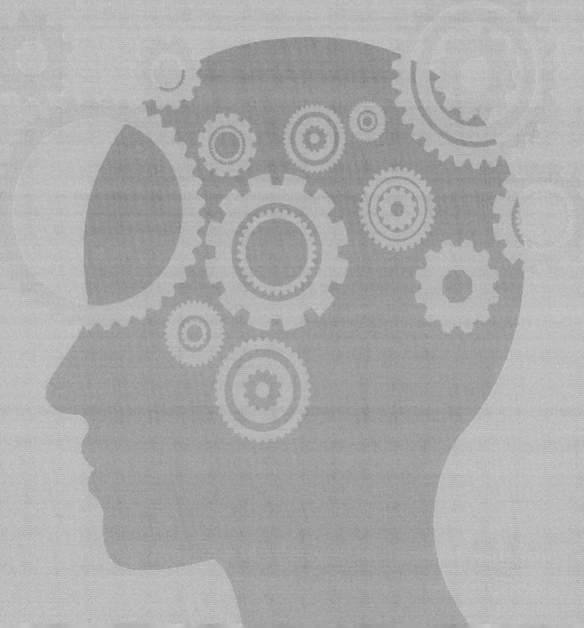

References

Bailey R (1995) *How to Empower People at Work*, Management Books 2000, Oxford.

Bailey R (2001) *NLP Counselling*, 2nd edn, Speechmark Publishing, Bicester, Oxon.

Bailey R (2010) *MasterStress*, Speechmark Publishing, Milton Keynes, Bucks.

Bailey R (2012) 'They just can't concentrate', Presentation, Shapwick School, Somerset.

Bailey R (2013) *Taming the Tiger: The A–Z of Managing Stress*, Personal Excellence Publications, Pilton, Somerset.

Bailey R & Brown E (2012) *Psychological Forum*, Elvie Brown Associates, Shepton Mallet, Somerset.

Bailey R & Brown E (2013) *The Concentration Assessment Profile (CAP)*, Speechmark Publishing, Milton Keynes, Bucks.

Bailey R & Clarke M (1989) *Stress and Coping in Nursing*, Chapman & Hall, London.

Best JB (1955) *Cognitive Psychology*, 4th edn, West, St Paul, Minn.

Brown E & Bailey R (2011) *Psychological Forum*, Elvie Brown Associates, Shepton Mallet, Somerset.

Brown E & Bailey R (2012) *Understanding and Improving Concentration*, Presentation, Millfield School, Glastonbury.

Brown E & Bailey R (2013) *Reframing and Training Concentration*, SATIPS, Great Dunmow, Essex.

Campbell KL, Grady CL, Ng C & Hasher L (2012) 'Age differences in the frontoparietal cognitive control network: implications for distractibility', *Neuropsychologica*, 50, pp2212–23.

Craik FIM, Goron R, Naveh-Benjamin M & Anderson ND (1996) 'The effects of divided attention on encoding and retrieval processes in human memory', *Journal of Experimental Psychology*, 125, pp159–80.

Csikzentmihalyi , M (1991) *Flow*, Harper, New York.

Deci EL (1975) *Intrinsic Motivation*, Plenum, New York.

Deci EL & Porac J (1978) 'Cognitive evaluation theory and the study of human motivation', Lepper MR & Greene D (eds), *The Hidden Costs of Reward*, Erlbaum, Hillsdale, NJ.

De Mello A (1997) *Awareness*, Fount Paperbacks, New York.

Dumont TQ (2006) *The Power of Concentration*, BiblioBazaar, Charleston.

Fehemi L and Robbins J (2007) *The Open-Focus Brain*, Trueter Books, Boston, Mass.

Frith C (2007) *Making Up the Mind*, Blackwell Publishing, Oxford.

Glasser W (1985) *Control Theory*, Harper Collins, New York.

Glasser W (1990) *Control Theory in the Practice of Reality Therapy*, Harper, New York.

Goldinger, SD, Kleider, HM Azuma, T& Beike, DR (2003) '"Blaming the victim" under memory load', *Psychological Science*, 3, pp53–61.

Griffey H (2010) *The Art of Concentration*, Rodale, London.

Gunaratana BH (2002) *Mindfulness in Plain English*, Wisdom Publications, Boston, Mass.

Heider F (1958) *The Psychology of Interpersonal Relations*, Wiley, New York.

James W (1890) *Principles of Psychology*, Holt Rinehart & Winston, New York.

Kabat-Zinn J (2003) *Mindfulness Meditation: Cultivating the Wisdom of Your Body and Mind*, Simon & Schuster Audio, New York.

Kahneman D (1973) *Attention and Effort*, Prentice-Hall, Englewood Cliffs, NJ.

Kelly HH (1967) 'Attribution theory in social psychology', Levine D (ed), *Nebraska Symposium on Motivation Volume 150*, University of Nebraska, Lincoln.

Lazarus R (1966) *Psychological Stress and the Coping Process*, McGraw-Hill, New York.

Lezak MD, Howieson DB & Loring DW (2004) *Neuropsychological Assessment*, Oxford University Press, Oxford.

Moran AP (2004) *The Psychology of Concentration in Sport Performers: A Cognitive Analysis*, Psychology Press, Hove, Sussex.

Moray N (1969) *Attention: Selective Processes in Vision and Hearing*, Hutchinson Educational, London.

Neisser U (1967) *Cognitive Psychology*, Appleton-Century-Crofts, New York.

Neisser U (1976) *Cognition and Reality*, WH Freeman, San Francisco, Calif.

Perlmutter LC & Chan F (1983) 'Does control of the environment enhance the perception of control?', *Motivation and Emotion*, 7, pp345–55.

Perlmutter LC & Monty RA (1977) 'The importance of perceived control: fact or fantasy?', *American Scientist*, 65, pp759–65.

Petri HL (1996) *Motivation*, 4th edn, Brooks/Cole Publishing Co., Pacific Grove, Calif.

Rogers C (1969) *Freedom to Learn*, Charles Merrill Publishing, Columbus, Ohio.

Rogers C (1986) *On Becoming a Person*, Constable, London.

Rossi L (1993) *The Psychobiology of Mind–Body Healing*, Norton, New York.

Sadhu M (2004) *Concentration: A Guide to Mental Mastery*, Aeon Books, London.

Seligman MEP (2004) *Authentic Happiness*, Nicholas Brealey Publishing, London.

Selye H (1979) 'The stress concept and some of its implications', Hamilton V & Warburton DM (eds), *Human Stress and Cognition: An Information Processing Approach*, Wiley, New York.

Thouless RH (1971) *Straight and Crooked Thinking*, Pan Books, London..

Treisman AM (1960) 'Contextual issues in selective listening', *Quarterly Journal of Experimental Psychology*, 12, pp212–8.

Treisman AM (1964) 'Verbal cues, language and meaning in selective attention', *American Journal of Psychology*, 77, pp206–19.

Wegner DM (1994) 'Ironic process of mental control', *Psychological Review*, 101, pp34–52.

Wegner DM (1997) 'When the antidote is the poison: ironic mental control processes', *Psychological Science*, 8 (3), pp148–50.

Whitmore J (2009) *Coaching for Performance*, 4th edn, Nicholas Brealey Publishing, London.

Wilson K & Koran JH (2007) 'Attention during lectures: beyond ten minutes', *Teaching Psychology*, 34 (2), p285.

Zuckier H & Hagen JW (1978) 'The development of selective attention under distracting conditions', *Child Development*, 49, pp870–3.

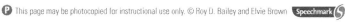